WHO Child Growth Standards

Growth velocity based on weight, length and head circumference

Methods and development

World Health Organization

Department of ... tion for ... ment

WHO Library Cataloguing-in-Publication Data

WHO child growth standards : growth velocity based on weight, length and head circumference : methods and development.

Coordinating team: Mercedes de Onis ... [et al.].

1.Anthropometry - methods. 2.Body size - standards. 3.Child development. 4.Growth. 5.Reference standards. 6.Nutrition assessment. I.de Onis, Mercedes. II.World Health Organization. Dept. of Nutrition for Health and Development.

ISBN 978 92 4 154763 5   (NLM classification: WS 103)

Members of the WHO Multicentre Growth Reference Study Group

Coordinating Team

Mercedes de Onis [Study Coordinator], Adelheid Onyango, Elaine Borghi, Amani Siyam, Alain Pinol (Department of Nutrition for Health and Development, World Health Organization).

Executive Committee

Cutberto Garza [Chair], Mercedes de Onis, Jose Martines, Reynaldo Martorell, Cesar G. Victora (up to October 2002), Maharaj K. Bhan (from November 2002).

Steering Committee

Coordinating Centre (WHO, Geneva): Mercedes de Onis, Jose Martines, Adelheid Onyango, Alain Pinol.

Investigators (by country): Cesar G. Victora and Cora Luiza Araújo (Brazil), Anna Lartey and William B. Owusu (Ghana), Maharaj K. Bhan and Nita Bhandari (India), Kaare R. Norum and Gunn-Elin Aa. Bjoerneboe (Norway), Ali Jaffer Mohamed (Oman), Kathryn G. Dewey (USA).

United Nations Agency Representatives: Cutberto Garza (UNU), Krishna Belbase (UNICEF).

Advisory Group

Maureen Black, Wm. Cameron Chumlea, Tim Cole, Edward Frongillo, Laurence Grummer-Strawn, Reynaldo Martorell, Roger Shrimpton, Jan van den Broeck. For the work presented in this document, Charlotte M Wright, John Himes, Huiqi Pan, Robert Rigby, Mikis Stasinopoulos and Stef van Buuren, participated in an advisory capacity.

Participating countries and investigators

Brazil: Cora Luiza Araújo, Cesar G. Victora, Elaine Albernaz, Elaine Tomasi, Rita de Cássia Fossati da Silveira, Gisele Nader (Departamento de Nutrição and Departamento de Medicina Social, Universidade Federal de Pelotas; and Núcleo de Pediatria and Escola de Psicologia, Universidade Católica de Pelotas).

Ghana: Anna Lartey, William B. Owusu, Isabella Sagoe-Moses, Veronica Gomez, Charles Sagoe-Moses (Department of Nutrition and Food Science, University of Ghana; and Ghana Health Service).

India: Nita Bhandari, Maharaj K. Bhan, Sunita Taneja, Temsunaro Rongsen, Jyotsna Chetia, Pooja Sharma, Rajiv Bahl (All India Institute of Medical Sciences).

Norway: Gunn-Elin Aa. Bjoerneboe, Anne Baerug, Elisabeth Tufte, Kaare R. Norum, Karin Rudvin, Hilde Nysaether (Directorate of Health and Social Affairs; National Breastfeeding Centre, Rikshospitalet University Hospital; and Institute for Nutrition Research, University of Oslo).

Oman: Ali Jaffer Mohamed, Deena Alasfoor, Nitya S. Prakash, Ruth M. Mabry, Hanadi Jamaan Al Rajab, Sahar Abdou Helmi (Ministry of Health).

USA: Kathryn G. Dewey, Laurie A. Nommsen-Rivers, Roberta J. Cohen, M. Jane Heinig (University of California, Davis).

Acknowledgements

The WHO Child Growth Standards were constructed by the Coordinating Team in the Department of Nutrition for Health and Development of the World Health Organization.

The Study Group is indebted to the parents, children and more than 200 field staff that participated in the WHO Multicentre Growth Reference Study. The generous contribution of many individuals that provided expertise and advice was also crucial to the development of the growth standards.

The project received funding from the Bill & Melinda Gates Foundation, the Netherlands Minister for Development Cooperation, the Norwegian Royal Ministry of Foreign Affairs, and the United States Department of Agriculture (USDA). Financial support was also provided by the Ministry of Health of Oman, the United States National Institutes of Health, the Brazilian Ministry of Health and Ministry of Science and Technology, the Canadian International Development Agency, the United Nations University, the Arab Gulf Fund for United Nations Development, the Office of the WHO Representative to India, and the WHO Department of Child and Adolescent Health and Development.

Contents

Figures

Appendix A3

Appendix C

Tables

Appendix A3

Appendix A4

Appendix A5

Appendix B

Appendix C

Glossary

BCPE	The Box-Cox power exponential distribution.
μ	The median of the Box-Cox power exponential distribution.
σ	The approximate coefficient of variation of the Box-Cox power exponential distribution — related to the variance.
ν	The power of the Box-Cox transformation (to the normal distribution) of the Box-Cox power exponential distribution - related to the skewness.
τ	The power exponential parameter of the Box-Cox power exponential distribution — related to the kurtosis.
λ	The power of the age (or starting weight) transformation.
δ	A constant value (delta) added to weight increments.
Box-Cox transformation	A power transformation to the normal distribution.
Coefficient of variation	The ratio of the standard deviation to the mean.
Cubic spline	A piecewise third-order polynomial function that passes through a set of m (or degrees of freedom) control points; it can have a very simple form locally, yet be globally flexible and smooth.
Cut-off	A designated limit beyond which a subject or observation is classified according to a pre-set condition.
Degrees of freedom (df)	The number of control points used to fit the cubic splines.
Kurtosis	An attribute of a distribution describing "peakedness". A high kurtosis portrays a distribution with fat tails in contrast to a low kurtosis, which portrays a distribution with skinny tails.
P-value	The probability of falsely rejecting the hypothesis being tested. In this report all p-values were compared to a level of significance set to 0.05.
Q-test	A statistical test which combines overall and local tests assessing departures from the normal distribution with respect to median, variance, skewness and kurtosis.
Skewness	A statistical term used to describe a distribution's asymmetry in relation to a normal distribution.
Standard deviation score (SD)	See z-score.
Worm plots	A set of detrended Q-Q plots — plots that compare the distribution of a given set of observations to the normal distribution.
Z-score	The deviation of an individual's value from the median value of a reference population divided by the standard deviation of the reference population (or transformed to normal distribution).

Executive summary

In 1993, the World Health Organization (WHO) undertook a comprehensive review of the uses and interpretation of anthropometric references. The review concluded that the National Center for Health Statistics (NCHS)/WHO growth reference, which had been recommended for international use since the late 1970s, did not adequately represent early childhood growth and that new growth curves were necessary. The World Health Assembly endorsed this recommendation in 1994. In response, the WHO Multicentre Growth Reference Study (MGRS) was implemented between 1997 and 2003 to develop international growth standards for children below 5 years of age. The MGRS is unique in that it was purposely designed to produce a standard by selecting healthy children from diverse ethnic backgrounds living under conditions likely to favour the achievement of their full genetic growth potential. Furthermore, the mothers of the children selected for the construction of the standards engaged in fundamental health-promoting practices, namely breastfeeding and not smoking. The first set of the WHO Child Growth Standards for attained growth based on length/height, weight and age was released in April 2006. The second complementary set, based on head and arm circumference and subscapular and triceps skinfolds, followed a year later.

A key component in the MGRS design was a longitudinal cohort of children who were examined in a sequence of 21 visits starting at birth and ending at 24 months of age. Such frequently collected and well-controlled data are highly unusual. A principal rationale for the MGRS longitudinal component was to allow for the development of growth velocity standards. The increments on which the velocity standards are based were calculated using the longitudinal sample of 882 children (428 boys and 454 girls) whose mothers complied fully with the MGRS infant-feeding and no-smoking criteria and completed the follow-up period of 24 months. The children were measured at birth; at weeks 1, 2, 4 and 6; monthly from 2–12 months; and bimonthly in the second year.

On the recommendation of a consultative expert group it was decided to develop velocity standards for the following anthropometric variables: weight (the most commonly used measurement and the most responsive to short-term influences), head circumference (the next most-used measurement in clinical settings), and length (potentially useful since stunting originates in the first two years of life, and early detection of changes in velocity may be beneficial for prevention). It was hypothesized that body mass index (BMI) velocity might be useful in predicting changes leading to extremes of adiposity. However, unreliability in BMI increments is a composite of measurement error from various sources. Moreover, BMI peaks during infancy and then drops through the second year. These characteristics make BMI velocity difficult to interpret, and there is little knowledge of its prognostic utility. Therefore, BMI velocity standards were not developed.

Another recommendation by the consultative expert group on the construction of the velocity curves was to explore other distributions in addition to the one used to construct the attained growth standards (the Box-Cox-power-exponential — BCPE). This investigation was carried out in an effort to identify the most appropriate methodology for handling anticipated negative increments specifically in relation to weight. The findings favoured the application of the BCPE distribution with some methodological adjustments only in the case of weight conditional on age. The steps followed to select the best models to fit the data for each indicator were comparable to those used to construct the attained growth standards.

Before the BCPE could be applied to the weight increments conditional on age, it was necessary to add a constant value, delta, to all weight increments to shift their distribution above zero. Afterwards, the predicted centiles were shifted down by the pre-added delta. By the MGRS design, the latest 3-month increment that could be calculated based on observed measurements was from age 11 to 14 months. The 3-month velocities were constructed for the full age range (birth to 24 months) using the parameter curves estimated for the 2-month (birth to 24 months), the 3-month (birth to 14 months) and the 4-month (birth to 24 months) intervals jointly in a cubic spline surface. All velocity standards required the modelling of skewness. In the interest of keeping the z-score calculation formula simple and considering the fact that adjustment for kurtosis had negligible impact on the final predicted centiles, it was decided not to fit kurtosis (i.e. models were restricted to the LMS class). The diagnostic tools used iteratively to detect possible model misfits and biases in the fitted curves included tests of local and global goodness of fit, such as Q-tests and worm plots. Patterns of differences between empirical and fitted centiles were also examined.

Following wide consultation with different potential users of these standards (e.g. paediatric endocrinologists, neonatologists, lactation counsellors, managers of child health programmes, and researchers), the increments presented in this report are those considered to be most useful clinically. The WHO velocity standards for weight are presented as 1-mo increments from birth to 12 months, and as 2- to 6-month incements from birth to 24 months. In addition, weight increments are presented from birth to 60 days in 1-week and 2-week intervals that coincide with the measurement schedule in the MGRS. The velocity standards for length are presented in 2- to 6-month increments from birth to 24 months. For head circumference, 2- and 3-month increments are presented from birth to 12 months, and 4- and 6-month increments from birth to 24 months. One-month increments for length and head circumference were not considered clinically useful as the measurement error over such a short period exceeds the 5th centile as early as 6 months of age. For similar reasons, the 2- and 3-month increments for head circumference go up to 12 months of age only. The overall choice of intervals is in line with those proposed by other authors. Electronic copies of the full set of velocity standards are available on the Web: www.who.int/childgrowth/en.

The intrinsic biological complexity of the dynamics of human growth makes the use and interpretation of the standards presented in this report more challenging than that of the attained growth standards. Growth progresses at a rapidly decelerating rate from birth, reaching a near-plateau by the end of the first year, and continues to taper off gently through the second year. This is the expected overall pattern of growth under conditions of adequate nutrition and psychosocial care. However, growth velocities of individual children are characterized by very high variability in consecutive growth intervals. It is not unusual for a child to grow at the 95th velocity centile one month and at the 20th the next while continuing to track on the attained weight-for-age chart. Correlations between subsequent increments are typically low; this reflects both a natural pattern of saltatory growth and possible catch-up or catch-down growth that contributes to overall narrowly canalized patterns in the attained growth trajectories of individual children.

The 1-, 2-, 3-, 4- and 6-month increment tables are independent of each other and the clinician should use the one that most closely approximates the interval over which the child is seen. For example, the centile corresponding to an increment between age 2 and 3 months is not associated with the centile corresponding to half of the increment in the 2-month interval between ages 1 and 3 months. This is because one cannot expect the growth rate in a given 2-month period, except perhaps at the median, to be the sum of the two corresponding 1-month intervals. With specific reference to weight, negative increments, which generally occur after 6 months of age, are captured in the lowest centiles. They coincide with the weaning period, when children are more exposed to food contamination, and when they become more active and start to explore their environment.

The tables of weight velocity from birth to 60 days present physiological weight losses that occur in the early postnatal period but are not usually included in available reference data. It was not possible to estimate from these data precisely when infants should recover their birth weight following weight loss that is common in the first few postnatal days. Net increments at the median (0 to 7 days) are positive for both boys and girls, suggesting that recovery of birth weight could be achieved in less than one week. Considering the 25th centile (0 g increment from birth to 7 days), the data suggest that 75% of newborns recover their birth weight by day 7. It is understood that recovery depends on what percentage of birth weight was lost and the successful initiation of lactation. However, rather than focus only on weight gain, it is important to adopt a holistic approach that looks at the child's overall health status and clinical signs, which are key to maintaining successful infant nutrition. This includes also assessing mother-child interaction, indicators of successful breastfeeding such as infant breastfeeding behaviour and the timing of stage II lactogenesis, and breastfeeding technique. Centiles are presented for both net increments and velocity in g/d. When mother-child dyads experience breastfeeding difficulties in the early postpartum period, lactation performance and weight gain are monitored every few days, hence increments per day are likely to be handier to use than weekly or fortnightly increments. However, even in the absence of such difficulties, visits to the clinic take place at random ages, and these daily increments offer a flexible option for evaluating growth over fractions of the tabulated time blocks.

Measurements of growth are subject to error from multiple sources. Faulty measurements can lead to grossly erroneous judgements regarding a child's growth. The accuracy of growth assessment is improved greatly if measurements are replicated independently and the values averaged. Although the high level of reliability achieved in the MGRS is unlikely to be reached in routine clinical measurement in primary health care settings, measurements need to be taken with reasonable care and accuracy as the calculation of increments involves two measurement errors.

Ideally, velocity assessment should be done at scheduled visits that coincide with the ages and intervals (1, 2, 3, 4 and 6 months) for which the centiles are presented. In practice, however, the timing of clinic visits is dictated by uncontrollable factors, and ingenuity will be called for in applying the standards. The discussion section of the report provides overall guidance on interpreting increments that are beyond the allowable range of variation around the intervals, or observed intervals that are on target (say exactly 2 months) but with starting and ending ages that do not coincide with those tabulated in the standards.

There are some fundamental differences between velocity and attained (distance) growth that affect how the increment standards should be used and interpreted. Chief among them is the lack of correlation between successive increments in healthy, normally growing children. For individual attained growth curves, the variability in successive z-scores tends to be minimal over short periods (there are high correlations between successive attained values). This "tracking" is not usually seen for successive individual growth velocities. In the WHO standards, the probability of two consecutive 1-month or 2-month weight increments falling below the 5th centile is 0.3%. If the 15th centile is chosen, this probability increases to only 2% and 1.8%, respectively. Normally growing children can have a very high z-score one month and a very low one the following month, or vice versa, without any underlying reason for concern. Thus, a single low value is not informative; only when velocities are repeatedly low should they cause concern. Nevertheless, very low z-score values, even if observed only once, should raise the question of whether there is underlying morbidity within the holistic clinical assessment of the child.

During periods of severe illness (e.g. prolonged diarrhoea) one would expect very low velocity followed by compensatory high velocity (catch-up). During catch-up growth, one would expect successive increments to be repeatedly in the higher ranges. An important difference with attained growth is that single extreme values of increments are comparatively less worrisome. Ultimately, growth velocity must always be interpreted in conjunction with attained growth, since the position on the attained growth chart is essential to interpreting the growth rate.

The velocity standards presented in this report provide a set of tools for monitoring the rapid and changing rate of growth in early childhood. Future research will need to determine what patterns of successive velocity thresholds over which specified intervals have the best diagnostic and prognostic validity for specific diseases.

1. INTRODUCTION

The WHO Multicentre Growth Reference Study (MGRS) was implemented between 1997 and 2003 to develop growth standards for children below 5 years of age. The MGRS collected primary growth data and related information from 8440 healthy breastfed infants and young children from diverse ethnic backgrounds and cultural settings (de Onis et al., 2004a). The first set of the WHO Child Growth Standards based on length/height, weight and age that describe the attained growth of healthy children was released in April 2006. The second complementary set, based on head and arm circumference and subscapular and triceps skinfolds, followed a year later (WHO Multicentre Growth Reference Study Group, 2006a; 2007). The standards are based on a prescriptive approach using well-defined criteria, rigorous data-collection methods, sound data-management procedures, and state-of-the art statistical methods (de Onis et al., 2004b; Borghi et al., 2006).

A key component in the MGRS design was a longitudinal cohort of children who were examined in a sequence of 21 visits starting at birth and ending at 24 months of age. Such frequently collected and well-controlled data are highly unusual, especially given the study's rigorous inclusion criteria (de Onis et al., 2004b). A principal rationale for the MGRS longitudinal component was to allow for development of velocity growth standards.

Proponents of the use of growth velocity consider it a superior quantitative measure of growth compared to attained size for age (Tanner, 1952; Roche and Himes, 1980; Baumgartner et al., 1986; Guo et al., 1991). They point out that, whereas pathogenic factors affect growth velocity directly, their impact on attained size becomes evident only after the altered rate of growth has had time to produce its result (Tanner, 1952). In other words, examining velocity should lead to earlier identification of growth problems than would the examination of attained growth only. Despite their hypothesized advantage, there are far fewer velocity references than there are for attained growth, in part due to scarcity of appropriate longitudinal datasets.

This report presents the WHO growth velocity standards and describes the methods used to construct the standards for weight conditional on age, weight conditional on age and birth weight, length conditional on age, and head circumference conditional on age. Strictly speaking, velocity is a change in value expressed in units per time period (e.g. g/time), while an increment is a change in value expressed in units (e.g. grams). Nevertheless, since the increments presented in this report refer to specific time periods (i.e. 1- to 6-month intervals), the terms velocity and increment will be used interchangeably.

As part of the preparatory work for the construction of the standards presented in this report, an advisory group met in March 2007 to review uses of growth velocity standards in clinical practice, public health programmes, and research settings and to discuss available strategies and related methods for the construction of the velocity standards. Two background documents were prepared to guide the advisory group's discussions, one on technical and statistical issues (Himes and Frongillo, 2007) and another on the presentation and application of such standards (Wright, 2007).

Among technical issues discussed, the first was whether to model increments (i.e. using measurements) or changes in z-scores. The complexity in applying growth velocity using available presentation formats associated with the z-score scale was recognized.

The second technical issue concerned which approach to statistical modelling to use for the increments, i.e. GAMLSS (Rigby and Stasinopoulos, 2005) or multi-level (ML) (Goldstein, 1986) modelling. The consensus was in favour of GAMLSS over ML modelling because it had been used more extensively in growth curve construction and its capabilities and associated diagnostic tests were better understood. Multi-level modelling was believed to be potentially extremely complex given the large number of growth intervals in the WHO standards data that would have to be modelled. In addition, use of the GAMLSS method as recommended by the background document on statistical issues (Himes and Frongillo, 2007) provided consistency with the methodology used to construct the WHO attained growth standards. Technical aspects regarding presentation and application included the choice of variables and intervals, and whether data should be displayed as tables or curves. The need for guidance on the use and interpretation of velocity standards was also recognized. It was decided to develop velocity standards for the following anthropometric variables: weight (the most commonly used measurement and the most responsive to short-term influences); head circumference (the next most-used measurement in clinical settings, mainly by neonatologists and others caring for infants); and length (potentially useful since stunting originates in the first two years of life, and detecting changes in velocity during this period may be beneficial in terms of prevention). It was hypothesized that BMI velocity might be useful in predicting changes leading to extremes of adiposity. However, unreliability in BMI increments is a composite of measurement error from various sources. Moreover, BMI peaks during infancy and then drops through the second year. These characteristics make BMI velocity difficult to interpret, and there is little knowledge of its prognostic utility. Therefore, BMI velocity standards were not developed. The final choice of variables (weight, length and head circumference) is similar to other published velocity references (Falkner, 1958; Tanner et al., 1966a, 1966b; Roche and Himes, 1980; Tanner and Davies, 1985; Baumgartner et al., 1986; Roche et al., 1989; Guo et al., 1991; van't Hof et al., 2000).

When selecting measurement intervals, account should be taken of the fact that the calculation of increments involves two measurement errors; hence data are usable only if the measurements are taken with reasonable care and accuracy. Measurement intervals should be wide enough that expected growth exceeds measurement error (Tanner, 1952; Cole, 1995; Himes, 1999). In some cases, velocity reference data (conditional on age) have been presented in yearly intervals (Tanner et al., 1966a; 1966b; Prader et al., 1989), usually from early childhood to early adulthood. However, such intervals cannot be used to detect nascent growth problems with a view to initiating timely corrective action. Falkner (1958) presented reference data for length, weight and head circumference in intervals ranging from three months in the first year to six months in the second year, and one interval from age 2 to 3 years. Baumgartner et al. (1986) published data for 6-month increments from birth to 18 years. Roche et al. (1989) presented centiles of monthly weight and length increments from the Fels Longitudinal sample (birth to 12 months). Two years later, Guo et al. (1991) published reference values of g/d or mm/d in variable (1- to 3-month) intervals. Following wide consultation with potential users of these standards (e.g. paediatric endocrinologists, neonatologists, lactation counsellors, managers of child health programmes, and researchers), the increments presented in this report are those considered to be the most useful clinically.

The WHO velocity standards for weight are presented in two output types. The main output concerns increments conditional on age, presented as 1-month intervals from birth to 12 months, and in 2- to 6-month intervals from birth to 24 months. The second output presents empirical centiles of increments from birth to 60 days in 1-week and 2-week intervals that coincide with the measurement schedule in the MGRS: birth to 7 days, and 7-14, 14-28, 28-42 and 42-60 days. These data are presented both as net increments in grams and as g/day velocities over each index period. It is expected that they will be especially useful for lactation management purposes during this critical period for establishing breastfeeding.

The velocity standards for length are presented in 2- to 6-month increments from birth to 24 months. For head circumference, 2- and 3-month increments are presented from birth to 12 months, and 4- and 6-month increments from birth to 24 months. We did not consider 1-month increments for length and head circumference to be clinically useful as the measurement error over such a short period exceeds the 5th centile as early as 6 months of age. For similar reasons, the 2- and 3-month increments for head circumference go up to 12 months of age only. The Technical Error of Measurement (TEM) in the longitudinal study of the MGRS was 0.38 cm for length and 0.24 cm for head circumference (WHO Multicentre Growth Reference Study Group, 2006b). Growth standards should allow for low velocities (e.g. 5th centile) to be detected with some certainty if they are to be clinically useful in detecting growth problems. The overall choice of intervals is supported by approaches suggested by other authors (Himes, 1999).

An important consideration regarding the presentation of standards relates to whether centiles are presented as curves or tabulated values. Curves for attained growth are commonly used to track individual growth patterns, but they cannot serve an equivalent purpose for growth velocity. High levels of intra-individual variation in velocity are normal, and it is not unusual for an infant whose increment at one interval was on the 5th centile to gain at the 75th centile during the next interval. Correlations between subsequent increments are typically low, reflecting a natural pattern of saltatory growth (Lampl et al., 1992) as well as possible catch-up or catch-down growth that contribute to overall narrowly canalized patterns in attained growth trajectories of individual children. For users habituated to attained growth curves, the interpretation of velocity curves presents a counter-intuitive logic: children are not expected to track on a fixed velocity curve (Healy et al., 1988) except perhaps in the median range (Tanner et al., 1966b). For example, a child whose weight velocity tracks on the 3rd centile from 5 to 16 years of age would be lighter at 16 years than a 5 year-old (Baumgartner et al., 1986). On the other hand, a child following the 97th centile from pre-school age would, by maturity, be pathologically enormous (Tanner et al., 1966b).

The lack of correlation between increments makes it difficult to define what constitutes a normal or abnormal sequence of increments, leading to the recommendation that velocity be examined always in conjunction with related measures of attained growth (Tanner, 1952). Different variants of charts combining the concepts of attained size and velocity have been developed and proposed for clinical use, particularly in the United Kingdom (Wright et al., 1994; Cole, 1997; Cole, 1998; Wright et al., 1998). However, those tools do not appear to have gained currency even when incorporated into computerized applications.

The models used in developing the WHO growth velocity standards produce centiles on a continuous scale, but the final centile values are presented in tabular format only for the specific age intervals described earlier. Graphic diagnostic outputs with point estimates linked as curves (not model-based curves) are presented throughout the report to facilitate comparisons between fitted and empirical centiles. Electronic copies of the full set of velocity standards are available on the Web: www.who.int/childgrowth/en. These standards provide a set of tools for monitoring the rapid and changing rate of growth in early childhood.

2. METHODOLOGY

2.1 Design of the WHO Multicentre Growth Reference Study

The MGRS (July 1997–December 2003) was a population-based study undertaken in Davis, California, USA; Muscat, Oman; Oslo, Norway; and Pelotas, Brazil; and in selected affluent neighbourhoods of Accra, Ghana and South Delhi, India. The MGRS protocol and its implementation in the six sites are described in detail elsewhere (de Onis et al., 2004a). Briefly, the MGRS combined a longitudinal component from birth to 24 months with a cross-sectional component of children aged 18–71 months. The longitudinal sample with visits planned at target ages allowed for the construction of growth velocity standards, which are the focus of this report. Mothers and newborns were screened and enrolled at birth and visited at home a total of 21 times on weeks 1, 2, 4 and 6; monthly from 2–12 months; and bimonthly in the second year. Data were collected on anthropometry, motor development, feeding practices, child morbidity, perinatal factors, and socioeconomic, demographic and environmental characteristics (de Onis et al., 2004b).

The study populations lived in socioeconomic conditions favourable to growth where mobility was low, ≥20% of mothers followed WHO feeding recommendations and breastfeeding support was available (de Onis et al., 2004b). Individual inclusion criteria were: no known health or environmental constraints to growth; mothers willing to follow MGRS feeding recommendations (i.e. exclusive or predominant breastfeeding for at least 4 months, introduction of complementary foods by the age of 6 months, and continued partial breastfeeding up to at least 12 months); no maternal smoking before and after delivery; single term birth; and absence of significant morbidity (de Onis et al., 2004c).

As part of the site-selection process in Ghana, India and Oman, surveys were conducted to identify socioeconomic characteristics that could be used to select groups whose growth was not environmentally constrained (Owusu et al., 2004; Bhandari et al., 2002; Mohamed et al., 2004). Local criteria for screening newborns, based on parental education and/or income levels, were developed from those surveys. Pre-existing survey data for this purpose were available from Brazil, Norway and the USA. The enrolment and baseline characteristics of the WHO Multicentre Growth Reference Study are described in detail elsewhere (WHO Multicentre Growth Reference Study Group, 2006c).

Term low-birth-weight (<2500 g) infants (2.3%) were *not* excluded. Since it is likely that in well-off populations such infants represent small but normal children, their exclusion would have artificially distorted the standards' lower centiles.

2.2 Anthropometry methods

Data collection teams were trained at each site during the study's preparatory phase, at which time measurement techniques were standardized against one of two MGRS anthropometry experts. During the study, bimonthly standardization sessions were conducted at each site. Once a year, the anthropometry expert visited each site to participate in these sessions (de Onis et al., 2004c). Results from the anthropometry standardization sessions have been reported elsewhere (WHO Multicentre Growth Reference Study Group, 2006b). For the longitudinal component of the study, screening teams measured newborns within 24 hours of delivery, and follow-up teams conducted home visits until 24 months of age (de Onis et al., 2004b).

The longitudinal component of the MGRS included data on weight, recumbent length (referred to subsequently as length) and head circumference, for which growth velocity standards are presented in this report. Observers working in pairs collected anthropometric data. Each observer independently measured and recorded a complete set of measurements, after which the two compared their readings. If any pair of readings exceeded the maximum allowable difference for a given variable (weight, 100 g; length, 7 mm; head circumference, 5 mm), both observers once again independently measured and recorded a second and, if necessary, a third set of readings for the variable(s) in question (de Onis et al., 2004b).

All study sites used identical measuring equipment. Instruments needed to be highly accurate and precise, yet sturdy and portable to enable them to be carried back and forth on home visits. Length was measured with the portable Harpenden Infantometer (range 30–110 cm, with digit counter readings precise to 1 mm). Portable electronic scales with a taring capability, calibrated to 0.1 kg (i.e. UNICEF Electronic Scale 890 or UNISCALE), were used to measure weight. A self-retracting, 0.7 cm-wide, flat metal tape with a blank lead-in strip (calibrated to 1 mm), was used to measure head circumference. Metal tapes were chosen because they are robust and accurate, and stay in a single plane around the head. They were replaced on a regular basis when the grading marks faded. Length and head circumference were recorded to the last completed unit rather than to the nearest unit. To correct for the systematic negative bias introduced by this practice, 0.05 cm (i.e. half of the smallest measurement unit) was added to each measurement before analysis. This correction did not apply to weight, which was rounded off to the nearest 100 g. Full details of the instruments used and how measurements were taken are provided elsewhere (de Onis et al., 2004c).

2.3   Sample description

A total of 1743 children were enrolled in the longitudinal sample, six of whom were excluded for morbidities affecting growth (4 cases of repeated episodes of diarrhoea, 1 case of repeated episodes of malaria, and 1 case of protein-energy malnutrition) leaving a sample of 1737 children (894 boys and 843 girls). Of these, the mothers of 882 children (428 boys and 454 girls) complied fully with the MGRS infant-feeding and no-smoking criteria and completed the follow-up period of 24 months (96% of compliant children completed the 24-month follow-up) (Table 1).

Table 1   Total sample and number of compliant children in the longitudinal component

Site	N	Compliant[a]		
		Boys	Girls	Total
Brazil	309	29	37	66
Ghana	328	103	124	227
India	301	84	89	173
Norway	300	75	73	148
Oman	291	73	76	149
USA	208	64	55	119
All	1737	428	454	882

[a] Compliant with infant-feeding and no-smoking criteria and completed the 24-month follow-up.

Based on the compliant children's data, 1-, 2-, 3-, 4- and 6-month increments were calculated for weight, length and head circumference. For weight, a total of 10 184 1-month increments (4909 for boys and 5275 for girls), 14 410 2-month increments (6950 for boys and 7460 for girls), 9294 3-month increments (4476 for boys and 4818 for girls), 12 690 4-month increments (6114 for boys and 6576 for girls) and 10 999 6-month increments (5299 for boys and 5700 for girls) were calculated. Shorter interval increments were also calculated between birth and two months following the MGRS design for use in lactation management programs (see section 3.2). For these shorter intervals, there were 2014 weight increments for boys and 2088 for girls. For length, a total of 14 520 2-month increments (7016 for boys and 7504 for girls), 9411 3-month increments (4545 for boys and 4866 for girls), 12 803 4-month increments (6183 for boys and 6620 for girls) and 11 097 6-month increments (5358 for boys and 5739 for girls) were calculated. For head circumference, a total of 14 517 2-month increments (7005 for boys and 7512 for girls), 9405 3-month increments (4536 for boys and 4869 for girls), 12 807 4-month increments (6178 for boys and 6629 for girls) and 11 100 6-month increments (5353 for boys and 5747 for girls) were calculated.

2.4 Data cleaning procedures and correction to target age

2.4.1 Data cleaning

Weight

Distributions of 1- and 2-month weight increments, not surprisingly, included negative increments (about 4.1% for the 1-month and 3.4% for the 2-month increments). In most cases, these were associated with reported morbidity and occurred mainly towards the end of Year 1 and in Year 2. Over 99.5% of negative increments were retained, as they are part and parcel of normal growth. Of the 16 403 weight values available, 57 (0.35%) with reported morbidity that entailed losses greater than 250 g per month were set to missing. Four additional weights (0.02%) without reported morbidity but with losses greater than 350 g per month in Year 1 or 1 kg per month in Year 2 were also set to missing. The threshold was set at approximately 10% of the median birth weight for the first year, and at about 10% of the median weight of a child at 12 months for the second year. In routine paediatric care, large weight losses, even in the absence of reported morbidity, are a sign of underlying problems (sub-clinical illness or psychosocial problems) that normally trigger diagnostic investigations. It is important to note that weights and not increments were excluded, which means that the large negative increments and the usually large positive increments immediately following them were both excluded.

Length and head circumference

In the case of length and head circumference no values were set to missing.

2.4.2 Correction to target age

The actual ages at which the measurements were made were at times delayed (or advanced on a few occasions) compared to the target ages. This resulted in some measurement intervals being either longer or shorter than planned by the MGRS design (e.g. 61 days for a 2-month interval). The data were corrected to target age as shown in Table 2.

Table 2   Maximum tolerable differences in days between planned and actual measurement ages.

Age range (months)	Maximum tolerable difference (Diff = Actual measurement age - target age[a])
0-6	± 3 days
6-12	± 5 days
12-24	± 7 days

[a] Target ages of the MGRS schedule were 0, 28, 61, 91, 122, 152, 183, 213, 244, 274, 304, 335, 365, 426, 487, 548, 609, 670, 731 days

The correction method was applied as follows:

- when the Diff was positive and greater than the tolerable difference indicated in Table 2, the measurement (i.e. weight, length or head circumference) corresponding to the target age was estimated by linear interpolation using measurements at the immediate previous visit and at the actual measurement age corresponding to the interval of interest. For example, if a visit was done at day 100 the weight measurement for the target visit age (91 days) was derived by interpolating between the weights at age 61 days and age 100 days.

- when the Diff was negative and greater in absolute value than the tolerable difference indicated in Table 2, the measurement (i.e. weight, length or head circumference) corresponding to the target age was estimated by linear interpolation using measurements at the actual age corresponding to the interval of interest and the immediate subsequent age that corresponded to the next planned visit. For example, for a visit at age 80 days, the estimated weight for age 91 days was based on weights at ages 80 and 122 days.

The correction to target age was applied to less than 10% of all measurements. The final numbers of observed increments used in the construction of the WHO child growth velocity standards are shown in Table 3.

Table 3   **Number of increments available for the construction of the WHO child growth velocity standards by sex and anthropometric indicator**

Indicator	Interval	Girls	Boys	Total
Weight	1-month	5242	4869	10 111
	2-month	7419	6889	14 308
	3-month	4789	4440	9229
	4-month	6537	6058	12 595
	6-month	5662	5247	10 909
Length	2-month	7504	7016	14 520
	3-month	4866	4545	9411
	4-month	6620	6183	12 803
	6-month	5739	5358	11 097
Head circumference	2-month[a]	5316	4947	10 263
	3-month	4869	4536	9405
	4-month	6629	6178	12 807
	6-month	5747	5353	11 100

[a] Number of available head circumference 2-month increments up to 14 months (see Chapter 5).

The fact that visits in the second year took place at 2-month intervals was a limitation when it came to constructing the 3-month velocity standards. The latest 3-month increment that could be calculated based on observed measurements was from age 11 to 14 months. The approach proposed to construct 3-month velocities for the full age range (birth to 24 months) was to use the parameter curves estimated for the 2-month (birth to 24 months), the 3-month (birth to 14 months) and the 4-month (birth to 24 months) intervals jointly in a cubic spline surface (described in section 2.5). In the case of head circumference, it was not necessary to apply this approach because the 3-month interval centiles were presented only up to age 12 months.

2.5   Statistical methods for constructing the growth velocity standards

The underlying methodology used for constructing the weight, length and head circumference velocity standards was the same used to construct the attained growth standards, i.e. the Box-Cox-power-exponential distribution (BCPE — Rigby and Stasinopoulos, 2004) with a cubic spline smoothing function. The growth curve fitting method and diagnostic tools used to select the best models for each of the indicators are described in detail in the report on the WHO child growth standards (WHO Multicentre Growth Reference Study Group, 2006a; 2007). In sum, the diagnostics included the Q-tests (Royston and Wright, 2000) and worm plots (van Buuren and Fredriks, 2001) for local and global goodness of fit. Patterns of differences between empirical and fitted centiles also were examined.

Weight velocities conditional on age required adjustment of the methodology to handle anticipated negative weight increments resulting from weight losses. The BCPE distribution is defined only on positive values. Distributions other than the BCPE were investigated for capability to handle negative increments. The two distributions that could be applied with no restrictions were the Sinh-arcsinh

(SHASH) distribution (Jones and Pewsey, 2008) and the skew exponential power (SEP) distribution (DiCiccio and Monti, 2004). Both distributions are recent methodologies that have not been extensively applied and tested on empirical data. However, both are available for application with the GAMLSS package (Stasinopoulos et al., 2004).

A few trials with the SHASH distribution were carried out using the 2-month weight increments sample. The modelling proved to be unstable. For example, in using the same approach as applied for the attained growth curves to select the best model, many of the models considered either failed to converge or did so only after 100 or more iterations. For the SEP distribution, also investigated using the 2-month weight increments sample, models would converge only for low degrees of freedom producing over-smoothed curves that fitted the data badly. Moreover, the SEP distribution requires numerical integration for the calculation of z-scores, which cannot be obtained without a computer. This would be a major drawback for the application of the growth velocity standards. Given the operational uncertainties around the application of these distributions and the poor results obtained when they were applied to the MGRS data, the decision was made to revert to the BCPE (which readily simplifies to the LMS method (Cole and Green, 1992) if no adjustment for kurtosis is necessary).

In some cases, there was residual kurtosis after adjusting for the skewness parameter. Conducted comparisons demonstrated that adjusting for kurtosis resulted in very slight shifts in the predicted centiles. In order to avoid having to apply the necessarily complicated resulting z-score calculation formula, the decision was made not to model kurtosis. The velocity data were thus fitted using the LMS method.

Before the BCPE could be applied to these data, it was necessary to add a constant value (termed delta, δ) to all weight increments to shift their distribution above zero. The BCPE was swift in fitting the data to predict centiles, which were then shifted downward by the pre-added delta. A similar procedure was applied in constructing the attained growth standards for length/height-for-age (WHO Multicentre Growth Reference Study Group, 2006a). To calculate z-scores, the delta value needs to be incorporated into the LMS formula. Delta should first be added to the child's increment and then the L, M and S values derived from the model fitted on the shifted observations should be used. When a child's increment is less than (-)delta (i.e. the increment is negative and its absolute value is greater than delta), the correction applied for the skewed attained growth standards beyond -3SD or +3SD applies (such an increment will always lie below -3SD). It was verified that, whereas the modelling process for each of these velocity standards was sensitive to the choice of delta, the final centile curves were practically unaffected and followed the empirical data closely.

For each interval for which the weight increment was modelled, a constant delta value was added at all ages, but it varied by sex for some of the intervals. The delta values were near the absolute value of the minimum observed increment at each interval. In the case of the 1-month interval, delta was 400 g for both sexes; for the 2-month interval, it was 600 g for both sexes; for the 4-month interval, it was 500 g for boys and 800 g for girls; and in the case of the 6-month interval, it was 350 g for boys and 450 g for girls. Exceptionally, three observed losses in the 4-month interval data for girls were between 600 g and 700 g. These were the result of smaller losses accumulated in two consecutive 2-month measurement intervals. Despite their magnitude, these negative increments were not excluded and in each case they were followed by compensatory large increments.

As noted in section 2.4, observed 3-month increments were available only up to 14 months of age. The approach proposed to construct 3-month velocities for the full age range (birth to 24 months) was to use parameter curves (L, M and S) estimated for the 2-month (birth to 24 months), the 3-month (birth to 14 months), and the 4-month (birth to 24 months) intervals jointly in a cubic spline surface.

The following steps were undertaken:

1. For weight, it was necessary to unify the delta across intervals for each sex (650 g for boys and 800 g for girls). The final BCPE model specifications for the 2- and 4-month intervals were re-applied to the data but using the unified delta values. For length, the final BCPE parameter estimates for the 2- and 4-month intervals were used.

2. For both length and weight 3-month intervals, the search for the best BCPE model was carried out using only observed increments (i.e. 1-4mo, 2-5mo,…,11-14mo). To minimize the right edge effect, parameter estimates up to 12 months only were used in the analyses described below.

3. L, M and S parameter estimates obtained in steps 1 and 2 were fed into a cubic spline fitting exercise (a surface fitting of the parameter as a function of age and interval) that was done for each of the parameters separately. The exception was the L values for length, which were estimated as constant values for both boys and girls. In this exercise, the ages corresponding to the intervals were shifted to their mid-point. The three parameters were each fitted on transformed age to the power 0.05 and, in addition, the natural logarithm transformation was applied to the S estimates (similar to GAMLSS modelling).

4. The estimation obtained from the cubic splines for each of the L, M and S parameters allowed the prediction of the 3-month velocity from birth to 24 months.

5. Finally, the predicted L, M and S values were used to construct the centile curves using the usual LMS formulae (including delta in the case of weight).

The Q-test results were interpreted and considered simultaneously with results of worm plots (van Buuren and Fredriks, 2001). On a few occasions, the two diagnostic tools indicated significant residual skewness for the selected models (e.g. girls' 2-month length velocity conditional on age). Worm plots were examined to detect any misfit of the median or the variance, or remaining skewness. Given that adjustment for kurtosis was never considered, there were some cases where the plots remained depicting non-flat worms (as S-shaped worms). It is worth mentioning that in all cases with significant residual skewness, increasing the number of degrees of freedom used to fit the parameter ν did not improve model adequacy. The selection of the model in those cases relied more on the goodness of fit when comparing fitted with predicted 3rd to 97th centiles. In sum, difficulties experienced in finding models of best fit, especially in adjusting for skewness, likely indicate that the smoothing curves cannot fully capture the inherent fluctuations across ages, rather than that the BCPE inadequately fits the increments at each age.

It is worth noting that in the case of velocities conditional on age, the variable age as used in the modelling exercise and subsequent diagnostic outputs refers to age in months at the end of the interval in question. For example, in the case of the 1-month weight velocity, an increment at age 5 months corresponds to the weight gain between ages 4 and 5 months. Prior to determining the best degrees of freedom for the parameter curves, a search was conducted for the best λ, the age-transformation power. For this, an arbitrary starting model (BCPE(x=age$^{\lambda}$, df(μ)=9, df(σ)=4, df(ν)=4, τ=2)) was used and the selection was based only on the global deviance values over a preset grid of λ values. The GAMLSS package (Stasinopoulos et al., 2004) was used to construct the growth standards.

3. CONSTRUCTION OF THE WEIGHT VELOCITY STANDARDS

3.1 Weight velocities conditional on age

The objective was to create sex-specific velocity curves for 1-, 2-, 3-, 4- and 6-month weight increments conditional on age. Tables generated from the 1-month increment curves contain estimated centiles for ages 0-1, 1-2, ..., 11-12 months; tables generated from the 2-month increment curves contain estimated centiles for ages 0-2, 1-3, ..., 22-24 months; tables generated from the 3-month increment curves contain estimated centiles for ages 0-3, 1-4, ..., 21-24 months; tables generated from the 4-month increment curves provide estimated centiles for ages 0-4, 1-5, ..., 20-24 months; and the tables from the 6-month increment curves provide estimated centiles for ages 0-6, 1-7, ..., 18-24 months.

3.1.1 1-month intervals

Boys

There were 4869 1-month weight increments for boys. The best value of the age-transformation power was $\lambda=0.05$. The search for the best $df(\mu)$ and $df(\sigma)$ followed, fixing $\lambda=0.05$, $\nu=1$ and $\tau=2$. The model with $df(\mu)=9$ and $df(\sigma)=4$ provided the smallest GAIC(3). The next step was to search for the best degrees of freedom to fit the parameter ν for skewness fixing $\tau=2$ and keeping the degrees of freedom for the previously selected μ and σ curves. The smallest GAIC(3) value corresponded to $df(\nu)=4$ and the model BCPE($x=age^{0.05}$, $df(\mu)=9$, $df(\sigma)=4$, $df(\nu)=4$, $\tau=2$) was further evaluated.

The diagnostic results are presented in Appendix A3, section A3.1a. The Q-test results (Table A3.1) and worm plots (Figure A3.1) from this model indicated residual skewness in only 1 out of 12 age groups. The overall Q-test p-values were all non-significant, indicating an adequate fit of the boys' 1-month weight increments. Figure A3.2 shows the fitted μ, σ and ν curves (dotted blue line) against their corresponding empirical estimates (points in red). There is no evidence of bias in any of the parameters. The next three figures (A3.3, A3.4 and A3.5) show no evidence of bias when comparing fitted against empirical centiles or centile residuals, except for a minor over-estimation of about 20 g in the 50th and 75th centiles.

Table 4 presents the predicted centiles for boys' 1-month weight velocities between birth and 12 months.

Girls

There were 5242 1-month weight increments for girls, eleven of which were excluded as outliers, leaving a final sample of 5231 observations for the modelling exercise. The best value of the age-transformation power was $\lambda=0.05$. The search for the best $df(\mu)$ and $df(\sigma)$ followed, fixing $\lambda=0.05$, $\nu=1$ and $\tau=2$. The model with $df(\mu)=13$ and $df(\sigma)=4$ provided the smallest GAIC(3). Yet the median fit for that model was under-smoothed compared to that of the boys and decreasing the $df(\mu)$ to 9 (the same as for the boys) resulted in a smoother curve. The next step was to search for the best degrees of freedom to fit the parameter ν for skewness fixing $\tau=2$ and keeping the degrees of freedom for the previously selected μ and σ curves. The smallest GAIC(3) value corresponded to $df(\nu)=1$ so the model BCPE($x=age^{0.05}$, $df(\mu)=9$, $df(\sigma)=4$, $df(\nu)=1$, $\tau=2$) was further evaluated.

The diagnostic results are presented in Appendix A3, section A3.1b. The Q-test results (Table A3.2) and worm plots (Figure A3.6) from this model indicated adequate fit as the overall Q-test p-values were non-significant at the 5% level. Figure A3.7 illustrates the fitting of parameters μ, σ and ν (dotted blue line) using the final model and their respective empirical estimates (points in red). No bias is observed for any of the parameters. Figures A3.8 and A3.9 show adequate fitting of centile curves.

Figure A3.10 depicts the distribution of the centile residuals, which indicate a slight over-estimation of the 75th centile (average of about 30 g) but no bias otherwise in any of the remaining centiles.

Table 5 presents the predicted centiles for girls' 1-month weight velocities between birth and 12 months.

3.1.2 2-month intervals

Boys

There were 6889 2-month weight increments for boys, seven of which were excluded as outliers, leaving a final sample of 6882 observations for the modelling exercise. The best value of the age-transformation power was $\lambda=0.05$. The search for the best df(μ) and df(σ) followed, fixing $\lambda=0.05$, $\nu=1$ and $\tau=2$. The model with df(μ)=12 and df(σ)=6 provided the smallest GAIC(3). The next step was to search for the best degrees of freedom to fit the parameter ν for skewness fixing $\tau=2$ keeping the degrees of freedom for the previously selected μ and σ curves. The smallest GAIC(3) value corresponded to df(ν)=3 and the model BCPE(x=age$^{0.05}$, df(μ)=12, df(σ)=6, df(ν)=3, $\tau=2$) was further evaluated.

The diagnostic results are presented in Appendix A3, section A3.2a. The Q-test results (Table A3.3) and worm plots (Figure A3.11) from this model indicated residual skewness in only 1 out of 17 age groups, and the overall Q-test p-values were non-significant at the 5% level. The fitted curves of the parameters μ, σ and ν seemed adequate when compared to the empirical values (Figure A3.12). The fitted centile curves and empirical centiles are shown in figures A3.13 and A3.14. Figure A3.15 shows the distribution of empirical minus fitted centile differences. There appears to be a slight but systematic under-estimation in the 25th centile, averaging about 25 g and countered by an equally slight over-estimation in the 75th centile.

Table 6 presents the predicted centiles for boys' 2-month weight velocities between birth and 24 months.

Girls

There were 7419 2-month weight increments for girls, ten of which were excluded as outliers, leaving a final sample of 7409 observations for the modelling exercise. The best value of the age-transformation power was $\lambda=0.05$. The search for the best df(μ) and df(σ) followed, fixing $\lambda=0.05$, $\nu=1$ and $\tau=2$. The model with df(μ)=12 and df(σ)=5 provided the smallest GAIC(3). The next step was to search for the best degrees of freedom to fit the parameter ν for skewness fixing $\tau=2$ and keeping the degrees of freedom for the previously selected μ and σ curves. The smallest GAIC(3) value corresponded to df(ν)=4 and the model BCPE(x=age$^{0.05}$, df(μ)=12, df(σ)=5, df(ν)=4, $\tau=2$) was further evaluated.

The diagnostic results are presented in Appendix A3, section A3.2b. The Q-test results (Table A3.4) and worm plots (Figure A3.16) from this model indicated residual skewness in only 1 out of 17 age groups and the overall Q-test p-values were non-significant at the 5% level. Figure A3.17 shows adequate fitting of the parameters μ, σ and ν with the respective sample estimates. Similar to the boys, comparisons between fitted and empirical centiles and centile residuals depict patterns of under-estimation (25th centile) and over-estimation (75th centile) of about 25 g (Figures A3.18 to A3.20).

Table 7 presents the predicted centiles for girls' 2-month weight velocities between birth and 24 months.

3.1.3 3-month intervals

Boys

There were 4440 3-month weight increments for boys, three of which were excluded as outliers, leaving a final sample of 4437 observations for the modelling exercise. The best value of the age-transformation power was $\lambda=0.05$. The search for the best df(μ) and df(σ) followed, fixing $\lambda=0.05$, $\nu=1$ and $\tau=2$. The model with df(μ)=8 and df(σ)=3 provided the smallest GAIC(3). The next step was to search for the best degrees of freedom to fit the parameter ν for skewness fixing $\tau=2$ and keeping the degrees of freedom for the previously selected μ and σ curves. The smallest GAIC(3) value corresponded to df(ν)=1 but df(ν)=2 yielded very similar GAIC(3) value and allowed the ν curve to closely follow the patterns observed for the 2- and 4-month intervals. Thus, for the benefit of jointly modelling parameter curves for the three intervals, the model BCPE(x=age$^{0.05}$, df(μ)=8, df(σ)=3, df(ν)=2, $\tau=2$) was selected to predict the boys' 3-month interval parameter curves up to age 12 months (see step 2 in section 2.5).

Those parameter estimates were joined to their equivalents obtained from the 2- and 4-month interval models (birth to 24 months) using the unified delta value (650 g) and a cubic spline surface was fitted for each parameter (L, M and S). The resulting predicted parameter estimates for interval 3-months (birth to 24 months) were used to construct the final centiles for boys.

The diagnostic results are presented in Appendix A3, section A3.3a. Figures A3.21 to A3.23 show minor bias (25 g on average) in the 10th and lower centiles (under-estimation) and a slight over-estimation in the 75th and 90th centiles (less than 50 g on average).

Table 8 presents the predicted centiles for boys' 3-month weight velocities between birth and 24 months.

Girls

There were a total of 4789 3-month weight increments for girls, seven of which were excluded as outliers, leaving a final sample of 4782 observations for the modelling exercise. The smallest global deviance value corresponded to the age-transformation power $\lambda=0.05$. The search for the best df(μ) and df(σ) followed, fixing $\lambda=0.05$, $\nu=1$ and $\tau=2$. The model with df(μ)=8 and df(σ)=4 provided the smallest GAIC(3). The next step was to search for the best degrees of freedom to fit the parameter ν for skewness fixing $\tau=2$ and keeping the degrees of freedom for the previously selected μ and σ curves. The smallest GAIC(3) value corresponded to df(ν)=4. The model BCPE(x=age$^{0.05}$, df(μ)=8, df(σ)=4, df(ν)=4, $\tau=2$) was selected to predict the girls' 3-month interval parameter curves up to age 12 months.

In accordance with step 3 of the methodology described in section 2.5, those parameter estimates were joined to their equivalents obtained from the 2- and 4-month interval models (birth to 24 months) using the unified delta value (800 g) and a cubic spline surface was fitted for each parameter (L, M and S). The resulting predicted parameter estimates for interval 3-months (birth to 24 months) were used to construct the final centiles for girls.

The diagnostic results are presented in Appendix A3, section A3.3b. The concordance between the predicted centiles and empirical values was evaluated by the comparisons in figures A3.24 to A3.26. Those show a slight over-estimation of about 50 g in the 75th and 90th centiles.

Table 9 presents the predicted centiles for girls' 3-month weight velocities between birth and 24 months.

3.1.4 4-month intervals

Boys

There were 6058 4-month weight increments for boys, two of which were excluded as outliers, leaving a final sample of 6056 observations for the modelling exercise. The best value of the age-transformation power was $\lambda=0.05$. The search for the best $df(\mu)$ and $df(\sigma)$ followed, fixing $\lambda=0.05$, $\nu=1$ and $\tau=2$. The model with $df(\mu)=11$ and $df(\sigma)=5$ provided the smallest GAIC(3). The next step was to search for the best degrees of freedom to fit the parameter ν for skewness fixing $\tau=2$ and keeping the degrees of freedom for the previously selected μ and σ curves. The smallest GAIC(3) value corresponded to $df(\nu)=6$ but with negligible difference from that yielded when $df(\nu)=5$. The model with the smaller $df(\nu)$ was selected, i.e. model BCPE($x=age^{0.05}$, $df(\mu)=11$, $df(\sigma)=5$, $df(\nu)=5$, $\tau=2$) and further evaluated.

The diagnostic results are presented in Appendix A3, section A3.4a. The Q-test results (Table A3.5) and worm plots (Figure A3.27) from this model indicated residual skewness in only 1 out of 15 age groups, with an overall Q-test p-value that was only marginally significant at the 5% level and thus the model was considered adequate. Figure A3.28 shows the fitted μ, σ and ν curves against their corresponding empirical estimates. Although there are notable fluctuations for the σ and ν parameters, the fitted curves seem adequate. The next three plots (figures A3.29 to A3.31) show no evidence of bias when comparing fitted against empirical centiles or centile residuals, except for an under-estimation in the 5th and 10th centiles, and an over-estimation in the 75th centile both less than 50 g.

Table 10 presents the predicted centiles for boys' 4-month weight velocities between birth and 24 months.

Girls

There were 6537 4-month weight increments for girls, four of which were excluded as outliers, leaving a final sample of 6533 observations for the modelling exercise. The best value of the age-transformation power was $\lambda=0.05$. The search for the best $df(\mu)$ and $df(\sigma)$ followed, fixing $\lambda=0.05$, $\nu=1$ and $\tau=2$. The model with $df(\mu)=9$ and $df(\sigma)=5$ provided the smallest GAIC(3). The next step was to search for the best degrees of freedom to fit the parameter ν for skewness fixing $\tau=2$ and keeping the degrees of freedom for the previously selected μ and σ curves. The smallest GAIC(3) value corresponded to $df(\nu)=5$ and the model BCPE($x=age^{0.05}$, $df(\mu)=9$, $df(\sigma)=5$, $df(\nu)=5$, $\tau=2$) was further evaluated.

The diagnostic results are presented in Appendix A3, section A3.4b. The Q-test results (Table A3.6) and worm plots (Figure A3.32) from this model indicated residual skewness in 3 out of 15 age groups. The overall Q-test p-value was marginally significant at the 5% level (p-value=0.0441). Figure A3.33 shows adequate fitting of the parameters μ, σ and ν with the respective sample estimates. Comparisons between fitted and empirical centiles and centile residuals depict patterns of under-estimation in the 10th and 97th centiles and over-estimation in the 75th centile by about 50 g (Figures A3.34 to A3.36). In sum, the selected model was considered adequate for constructing the 4-month velocity for girls.

Table 11 presents the predicted centiles for girls' 4-month weight velocities between birth and 24 months.

3.1.5 6-month intervals

Boys

There were 5247 6-month weight increments for boys, one of which was excluded as an outlier, leaving a final sample of 5246 observations for the modelling exercise. The best value of the age-transformation power was $\lambda=0.05$. The search for the best $df(\mu)$ and $df(\sigma)$ followed, fixing $\lambda=0.05$, $\nu=1$ and $\tau=2$. The model with $df(\mu)=10$ and $df(\sigma)=5$ provided the smallest GAIC(3). The next step was to search for the best degrees of freedom to fit the parameter ν for skewness fixing $\tau=2$ and keeping the degrees of freedom for the previously selected μ and σ curves. The smallest GAIC(3) value corresponded to $df(\nu)=3$. Thus the model BCPE($x=age^{0.05}$, $df(\mu)=10$, $df(\sigma)=5$, $df(\nu)=3$, $\tau=2$) was further evaluated.

The diagnostic results are presented in Appendix A3, section A3.5a. The Q-test results (Table A3.7) and worm plots (Figure A3.37) from this model indicated residual skewness in only 1 out of 13 age groups, with an overall Q-test p-value that was non-significant at the 5% level and thus the model was considered adequate. Figure A3.38 shows the fitted μ, σ and ν curves against their corresponding empirical estimates. There are some fluctuations for the parameter ν yet the fitted curve seems adequate. The next three plots (figures A3.39, A3.40 and A3.41) show a slight bias (of about 50 g) when comparing fitted against empirical centiles or centile residuals at the 5th and 10th centiles (under-estimation) and at the 75th and 90th centiles (over-estimation).

Table 12 presents the predicted centiles for boys' 6-month weight velocities between birth and 24 months.

Girls

There were 5662 6-month weight increments for girls, five of which were excluded as outliers, leaving a final sample of 5657 observations for the modelling exercise. The best value of the age-transformation power was $\lambda=0.05$. The search for the best $df(\mu)$ and $df(\sigma)$ followed, fixing $\lambda=0.05$, $\nu=1$ and $\tau=2$. The model with $df(\mu)=7$ and $df(\sigma)=5$ provided the smallest GAIC(3). The next step was to search for the best degrees of freedom to fit the parameter ν for skewness fixing $\tau=2$ and keeping the degrees of freedom for the previously selected μ and σ curves. The smallest GAIC(3) value corresponded to $df(\nu)=4$ and the model BCPE($x=age^{0.05}$, $df(\mu)=7$, $df(\sigma)=5$, $df(\nu)=4$, $\tau=2$) was further evaluated.

The diagnostic results are presented in Appendix A3, section A3.5b. The Q-test results (Table A3.8) and worm plots (Figure A3.42) from this model indicated residual skewness in 2 out of 13 age groups. The overall Q-test p-value for this parameter was marginally significant at the 5% level (p-value=0.0448). Figure A3.43 shows adequate fitting of the parameters μ, σ and ν with the respective sample estimates. Comparisons between fitted and empirical centiles and centile residuals depict patterns of under-estimation in the 5th and 10th centiles by less than 50 g and over-estimation in the 75th and 90th centiles by about 50 g (Figures A3.44 to A3.46). In sum, the selected model was considered adequate for constructing the 6-month velocity for girls.

Table 13 presents the predicted centiles for girls' 6-month weight velocities between birth and 24 months.

Table 4   Boys 1-month weight increments (g)

Interval	L[a]	M[a]	S[a]	δ	1st	3rd	5th	15th	25th	50th	75th	85th	95th	97th	99th
0-4 wks	1.3828	1423.0783	0.22048	400	182	369	460	681	805	1023	1229	1336	1509	1575	1697
4 wks-2 mo	0.7241	1596.3470	0.19296	400	528	648	713	886	992	1196	1408	1524	1724	1803	1955
2-3 mo	0.6590	1215.3989	0.19591	400	307	397	446	577	658	815	980	1071	1228	1290	1410
3-4 mo	0.7003	1017.0488	0.20965	400	160	241	285	403	476	617	764	845	985	1041	1147
4-5 mo	0.7419	921.6249	0.22790	400	70	150	194	311	383	522	666	746	883	937	1041
5-6 mo	0.7668	822.1842	0.24854	400	-17	61	103	217	287	422	563	640	773	826	927
6-7 mo	0.7688	756.5306	0.26783	400	-76	0	42	154	223	357	496	573	706	758	859
7-8 mo	0.7624	715.6257	0.28677	400	-118	-43	-1	111	181	316	457	535	671	724	827
8-9 mo	0.7620	684.7459	0.30439	400	-153	-77	-36	77	148	285	429	508	646	701	806
9-10 mo	0.7659	658.5809	0.32154	400	-183	-108	-66	48	120	259	405	486	627	683	790
10-11 mo	0.7713	643.4374	0.33882	400	-209	-132	-89	27	100	243	394	478	623	680	791
11-12 mo	0.7761	639.4743	0.35502	400	-229	-150	-106	15	91	239	397	484	635	695	811

Interval	L[a]	M[a]	S[a]	δ	-3SD	-2SD	-1SD	Median	1SD	2SD	3SD
0-4 wks	1.3828	1423.0783	0.22048	400	-160	321	694	1023	1325	1608	1876
4 wks-2 mo	0.7241	1596.3470	0.19296	400	354	615	897	1196	1512	1844	2189
2-3 mo	0.6590	1215.3989	0.19591	400	178	372	585	815	1061	1322	1597
3-4 mo	0.7003	1017.0488	0.20965	400	44	219	411	617	837	1069	1313
4-5 mo	0.7419	921.6249	0.22790	400	-45	128	318	522	738	965	1202
5-6 mo	0.7668	822.1842	0.24854	400	-128	40	224	422	632	853	1083
6-7 mo	0.7688	756.5306	0.26783	400	-183	-21	161	357	565	785	1014
7-8 mo	0.7624	715.6257	0.28677	400	-223	-63	118	316	528	752	987
8-9 mo	0.7620	684.7459	0.30439	400	-256	-98	84	285	500	729	969
9-10 mo	0.7659	658.5809	0.32154	400	-286	-128	55	259	478	711	956
10-11 mo	0.7713	643.4374	0.33882	400	-312	-153	34	243	469	710	963
11-12 mo	0.7761	639.4743	0.35502	400	-333	-172	22	239	475	726	990

[a] The L, M, S values provided are estimated based on the modelling of the shifted observations (i.e. by the addition of delta to the actual increment) which explains the difference (equals to delta) in value between the "M" and the 50th centile (or Median) values.

Table 5 Girls 1-month weight increments (g)

Interval	Lª	Mª	S	δ	1st	3rd	5th	15th	25th	50th	75th	85th	95th	97th	99th
0-4 wks	0.7781	1279.4834	0.21479	400	280	388	446	602	697	879	1068	1171	1348	1418	1551
4 wks-2 mo	0.7781	1411.1075	0.19384	400	410	519	578	734	829	1011	1198	1301	1476	1545	1677
2-3 mo	0.7781	1118.0098	0.19766	400	233	321	369	494	571	718	869	952	1094	1150	1256
3-4 mo	0.7781	984.8825	0.20995	400	133	214	259	376	448	585	726	804	937	990	1090
4-5 mo	0.7781	888.9803	0.22671	400	51	130	172	286	355	489	627	703	833	885	983
5-6 mo	0.7781	801.3910	0.24596	400	-24	52	93	203	271	401	537	611	739	790	886
6-7 mo	0.7781	744.3023	0.26515	400	-79	-4	37	146	214	344	480	555	684	734	832
7-8 mo	0.7781	710.6923	0.28409	400	-119	-44	-2	109	178	311	450	526	659	711	811
8-9 mo	0.7781	672.6072	0.30106	400	-155	-81	-40	70	139	273	412	489	623	675	776
9-10 mo	0.7781	644.6032	0.31676	400	-184	-110	-70	41	110	245	385	464	598	652	754
10-11 mo	0.7781	633.2166	0.33208	400	-206	-131	-89	24	95	233	378	459	598	653	759
11-12 mo	0.7781	631.7383	0.34627	400	-222	-145	-102	15	88	232	383	467	612	670	781

Interval	Lª	Mª	Sª	δ	-3SD	-2SD	-1SD	Median	1SD	2SD	3SD
0-4 wks	0.7781	1279.4834	0.21479	400	123	358	611	879	1161	1453	1757
4 wks-2 mo	0.7781	1411.1075	0.19384	400	251	490	744	1011	1290	1580	1880
2-3 mo	0.7781	1118.0098	0.19766	400	105	297	502	718	944	1178	1421
3-4 mo	0.7781	984.8825	0.20995	400	14	192	383	585	796	1016	1244
4-5 mo	0.7781	888.9803	0.22671	400	-62	108	293	489	695	911	1134
5-6 mo	0.7781	801.3910	0.24596	400	-132	31	210	401	604	815	1036
6-7 mo	0.7781	744.3023	0.26515	400	-185	-24	153	344	547	760	982
7-8 mo	0.7781	710.6923	0.28409	400	-224	-64	116	311	519	738	967
8-9 mo	0.7781	672.6072	0.30106	400	-259	-101	77	273	482	702	933
9-10 mo	0.7781	644.6032	0.31676	400	-286	-131	48	245	456	679	913
10-11 mo	0.7781	633.2166	0.33208	400	-307	-151	31	233	451	682	924
11-12 mo	0.7781	631.7383	0.34627	400	-324	-166	22	232	458	699	953

ª The L, M, S values provided are estimated based on the modelling of the shifted observations (i.e. by the addition of delta to the actual increment) which explains the difference (equals to delta) in value between the "M" and the 50ᵗʰ centile (or Median) values.

Table 6   Boys 2-month weight increments (g)

Interval	L[a]	M[a]	S[a]	δ	1st	3rd	5th	15th	25th	50th	75th	85th	95th	97th	99th
0-2 mo	0.7188	2815.6120	0.17422	600	1144	1338	1443	1720	1890	2216	2552	2737	3054	3179	3418
1-3 mo	0.6464	2592.0761	0.17025	600	1040	1211	1303	1549	1701	1992	2296	2463	2753	2868	3088
2-4 mo	0.6071	2038.1036	0.17559	600	675	810	884	1081	1202	1438	1685	1822	2059	2154	2336
3-5 mo	0.5915	1744.8197	0.18708	600	455	576	642	820	930	1145	1371	1496	1715	1802	1970
4-6 mo	0.5891	1541.3670	0.20130	600	291	404	466	634	738	941	1156	1277	1486	1569	1731
5-7 mo	0.5954	1377.6979	0.21318	600	165	271	330	487	585	778	982	1096	1294	1374	1528
6-8 mo	0.6088	1272.5277	0.22426	600	79	182	238	390	486	673	871	982	1175	1252	1402
7-9 mo	0.6270	1201.4599	0.23472	600	16	117	172	323	417	601	797	907	1098	1174	1322
8-10 mo	0.6486	1143.8903	0.24611	600	-41	60	115	266	360	544	739	848	1039	1115	1261
9-11 mo	0.6725	1101.6312	0.25918	600	-92	10	67	219	315	502	700	810	1003	1079	1227
10-12 mo	0.6959	1077.9049	0.27217	600	-132	-28	30	187	286	478	681	795	992	1070	1221
11-13 mo	0.7191	1057.9071	0.28462	600	-169	-62	-2	159	260	458	666	782	984	1064	1218
12-14 mo	0.7399	1037.0541	0.29479	600	-202	-92	-31	133	236	437	648	766	969	1050	1206
13-15 mo	0.7597	1014.1850	0.30285	600	-230	-119	-58	109	212	414	626	744	947	1028	1183
14-16 mo	0.7771	1000.5821	0.30864	600	-250	-138	-75	93	197	401	614	731	935	1016	1170
15-17 mo	0.7929	999.4661	0.31290	600	-262	-148	-84	87	193	399	615	734	939	1020	1176
16-18 mo	0.8078	1000.9680	0.31615	600	-272	-155	-90	84	192	401	619	739	945	1027	1183
17-19 mo	0.8210	998.4215	0.31858	600	-281	-162	-97	79	188	398	617	737	944	1025	1181
18-20 mo	0.8335	992.8040	0.32058	600	-291	-170	-104	73	182	393	611	731	937	1018	1173
19-21 mo	0.8447	986.9799	0.32222	600	-299	-178	-111	67	176	387	605	725	929	1010	1164
20-22 mo	0.8554	981.7965	0.32377	600	-307	-185	-118	61	171	382	599	719	923	1003	1156
21-23 mo	0.8655	978.4016	0.32529	600	-314	-191	-123	57	167	378	596	715	919	999	1151
22-24 mo	0.8748	976.3696	0.32673	600	-320	-196	-128	53	164	376	594	713	917	997	1149

[a] The L, M, S values provided are estimated based on the modelling of the shifted observations (i.e. by the addition of delta to the actual increment) which explains the difference (equals to delta) in value between the "M" and the 50th centile values.

Table 6   Boys 2-month weight increments (g) - *continued*

Interval	L[a]	M[a]	S[a]	δ	-3SD	-2SD	-1SD	Median	+1SD	+2SD	+3SD
0-2 mo	0.7188	2815.6120	0.17422	600	862	1285	1737	2216	2718	3243	3788
1-3 mo	0.6464	2592.0761	0.17025	600	795	1165	1564	1992	2446	2926	3430
2-4 mo	0.6071	2038.1036	0.17559	600	480	773	1093	1438	1808	2202	2619
3-5 mo	0.5915	1744.8197	0.18708	600	282	543	831	1145	1484	1846	2233
4-6 mo	0.5891	1541.3670	0.20130	600	131	373	644	941	1264	1612	1984
5-7 mo	0.5954	1377.6979	0.21318	600	16	242	497	778	1084	1414	1769
6-8 mo	0.6088	1272.5277	0.22426	600	-64	154	400	673	970	1292	1636
7-9 mo	0.6270	1201.4599	0.23472	600	-126	89	332	601	896	1213	1553
8-10 mo	0.6486	1143.8903	0.24611	600	-181	32	275	544	837	1153	1491
9-11 mo	0.6725	1101.6312	0.25918	600	-233	-18	229	502	799	1119	1459
10-12 mo	0.6959	1077.9049	0.27217	600	-278	-56	197	478	783	1110	1458
11-13 mo	0.7191	1057.9071	0.28462	600	-318	-91	169	458	771	1105	1459
12-14 mo	0.7399	1037.0541	0.29479	600	-353	-122	144	437	754	1092	1448
13-15 mo	0.7597	1014.1850	0.30285	600	-383	-149	119	414	732	1069	1424
14-16 mo	0.7771	1000.5821	0.30864	600	-405	-168	103	401	719	1057	1410
15-17 mo	0.7929	999.4661	0.31290	600	-421	-179	98	399	722	1061	1416
16-18 mo	0.8078	1000.9680	0.31615	600	-434	-187	95	401	726	1068	1424
17-19 mo	0.8210	998.4215	0.31858	600	-446	-195	90	398	725	1067	1422
18-20 mo	0.8335	992.8040	0.32058	600	-457	-203	84	393	719	1059	1412
19-21 mo	0.8447	986.9799	0.32222	600	-467	-211	78	387	712	1051	1401
20-22 mo	0.8554	981.7965	0.32377	600	-477	-218	72	382	707	1044	1391
21-23 mo	0.8655	978.4016	0.32529	600	-486	-224	68	378	703	1039	1385
22-24 mo	0.8748	976.3696	0.32673	600	-495	-230	65	376	701	1037	1382

[a] The L, M, S values provided are estimated based on the modelling of the shifted observations (i.e. by the addition of delta to the actual increment) which explains the difference (equals to delta) in value between the "M" and the Median values.

Table 7   Girls 2-month weight increments (g)

Interval	L[a]	M[a]	S[a]	δ	1st	3rd	5th	15th	25th	50th	75th	85th	95th	97th	99th
0-2 mo	0.4599	2497.0406	0.18000	600	968	1128	1216	1455	1604	1897	2210	2386	2696	2820	3062
1-3 mo	0.3294	2314.2285	0.17612	600	890	1030	1107	1317	1450	1714	2000	2163	2452	2569	2799
2-4 mo	0.3128	1907.0116	0.17761	600	625	740	804	978	1088	1307	1545	1681	1922	2020	2213
3-5 mo	0.3560	1673.5778	0.18421	600	451	556	615	773	874	1074	1290	1413	1632	1720	1894
4-6 mo	0.4264	1482.7466	0.19524	600	295	395	450	600	695	883	1085	1200	1403	1486	1646
5-7 mo	0.5002	1342.3734	0.20864	600	170	267	321	468	560	742	938	1048	1243	1321	1473
6-8 mo	0.5699	1251.4869	0.22315	600	76	175	229	377	469	651	846	955	1147	1223	1372
7-9 mo	0.6268	1181.4135	0.23586	600	3	103	157	306	399	581	775	883	1072	1147	1293
8-10 mo	0.6730	1116.8192	0.24680	600	-59	40	95	243	336	517	708	814	999	1073	1215
9-11 mo	0.7102	1078.3961	0.25656	600	-104	-3	53	203	297	478	670	776	960	1033	1174
10-12 mo	0.7382	1058.4112	0.26494	600	-135	-31	26	179	274	458	652	759	944	1018	1159
11-13 mo	0.7605	1040.8737	0.27292	600	-163	-57	1	157	254	441	637	745	932	1005	1147
12-14 mo	0.7762	1027.9459	0.28011	600	-185	-78	-19	140	238	428	626	736	924	999	1142
13-15 mo	0.7864	1019.6870	0.28705	600	-204	-95	-35	127	227	420	621	732	924	999	1144
14-16 mo	0.7913	1016.4898	0.29343	600	-219	-108	-47	118	220	416	622	735	930	1007	1154
15-17 mo	0.7922	1017.5335	0.29961	600	-231	-118	-55	112	216	418	627	743	943	1021	1172
16-18 mo	0.7902	1017.2241	0.30592	600	-243	-128	-64	106	212	417	631	750	954	1035	1189
17-19 mo	0.7866	1012.8511	0.31201	600	-255	-139	-75	97	205	413	631	751	959	1041	1199
18-20 mo	0.7827	1007.2711	0.31824	600	-267	-151	-86	88	196	407	628	751	962	1046	1206
19-21 mo	0.7795	1001.8324	0.32415	600	-279	-162	-97	79	188	402	626	750	965	1050	1213
20-22 mo	0.7771	993.3265	0.33014	600	-291	-174	-109	67	178	393	620	745	963	1049	1214
21-23 mo	0.7755	980.7096	0.33605	600	-305	-189	-124	53	164	381	608	735	954	1040	1207
22-24 mo	0.7743	967.2057	0.34166	600	-318	-202	-137	39	150	367	596	723	942	1029	1197

[a] The L, M, S values provided are estimated based on the modelling of the shifted observations (i.e. by the addition of delta to the actual increment) which explains the difference (equals to delta) in value between the "M" and the 50th centile values.

Table 7   Girls 2-month weight increments (g) - *continued*

Interval	L[a]	M[a]	S[a]	δ	-3SD	-2SD	-1SD	Median	+1SD	+2SD	+3SD
0-2 mo	0.4599	2497.0406	0.18000	600	742	1085	1469	1897	2368	2884	3445
1-3 mo	0.3294	2314.2285	0.17612	600	695	991	1330	1714	2146	2630	3167
2-4 mo	0.3128	1907.0116	0.17761	600	465	709	989	1307	1667	2071	2522
3-5 mo	0.3560	1673.5778	0.18421	600	304	528	783	1074	1400	1766	2172
4-6 mo	0.4264	1482.7466	0.19524	600	156	367	609	883	1189	1528	1901
5-7 mo	0.5002	1342.3734	0.20864	600	34	241	477	742	1037	1361	1714
6-8 mo	0.5699	1251.4869	0.22315	600	-61	148	386	651	944	1263	1607
7-9 mo	0.6268	1181.4135	0.23586	600	-136	75	315	581	872	1186	1522
8-10 mo	0.6730	1116.8192	0.24680	600	-199	13	253	517	803	1110	1437
9-11 mo	0.7102	1078.3961	0.25656	600	-246	-30	212	478	765	1070	1393
10-12 mo	0.7382	1058.4112	0.26494	600	-280	-60	188	458	748	1055	1378
11-13 mo	0.7605	1040.8737	0.27292	600	-311	-86	167	441	734	1043	1367
12-14 mo	0.7762	1027.9459	0.28011	600	-336	-107	150	428	724	1037	1363
13-15 mo	0.7864	1019.6870	0.28705	600	-358	-125	137	420	721	1038	1368
14-16 mo	0.7913	1016.4898	0.29343	600	-375	-138	128	416	723	1046	1383
15-17 mo	0.7922	1017.5335	0.29961	600	-389	-149	123	418	731	1062	1406
16-18 mo	0.7902	1017.2241	0.30592	600	-402	-159	117	417	738	1076	1428
17-19 mo	0.7866	1012.8511	0.31201	600	-414	-171	108	413	739	1083	1443
18-20 mo	0.7827	1007.2711	0.31824	600	-426	-183	99	407	738	1088	1455
19-21 mo	0.7795	1001.8324	0.32415	600	-438	-194	89	402	738	1093	1466
20-22 mo	0.7771	993.3265	0.33014	600	-450	-207	78	393	733	1093	1471
21-23 mo	0.7755	980.7096	0.33605	600	-462	-221	64	381	722	1085	1466
22-24 mo	0.7743	967.2057	0.34166	600	-474	-234	50	367	710	1074	1457

[a] The L, M, S values provided are estimated based on the modelling of the shifted observations (i.e. by the addition of delta to the actual increment) which explains the difference (equals to delta) in value between the "M" and the Median values.

Table 8   Boys 3-month weight increments (g)

Interval	L[a]	M[a]	S[a]	δ	1st	3rd	5th	15th	25th	50th	75th	85th	95th	97th	99th
0-3 mo	0.6854	3638.8730	0.15801	650	1733	1960	2083	2409	2608	2989	3383	3600	3972	4119	4401
1-4 mo	0.6503	3215.1010	0.16539	650	1415	1621	1733	2031	2214	2565	2931	3132	3480	3618	3882
2-5 mo	0.5884	2661.5629	0.17708	650	1011	1187	1284	1542	1702	2012	2337	2518	2833	2958	3199
3-6 mo	0.5368	2231.9042	0.18850	650	704	856	940	1166	1307	1582	1874	2038	2323	2438	2659
4-7 mo	0.4999	1939.0717	0.19877	650	496	632	707	910	1038	1289	1558	1709	1975	2082	2289
5-8 mo	0.4819	1745.5952	0.20848	650	355	480	550	739	859	1096	1350	1494	1748	1850	2049
6-9 mo	0.4866	1611.6464	0.21853	650	249	369	436	618	733	962	1208	1348	1595	1694	1888
7-10 mo	0.5135	1514.8958	0.22940	650	162	280	346	526	639	865	1108	1246	1489	1587	1778
8-11 mo	0.5582	1442.6013	0.24108	650	86	205	271	452	567	793	1036	1173	1414	1511	1700
9-12 mo	0.6092	1387.8840	0.25261	650	21	142	210	393	509	738	982	1120	1360	1457	1644
10-13 mo	0.6580	1346.3553	0.26315	650	-35	90	159	347	465	696	942	1080	1320	1416	1602
11-14 mo	0.7000	1314.9304	0.27214	650	-80	48	119	310	430	665	913	1051	1291	1387	1571
12-15 mo	0.7323	1291.3726	0.27922	650	-115	16	88	283	404	641	891	1029	1269	1364	1547
13-16 mo	0.7550	1273.8860	0.28446	650	-141	-8	65	263	385	624	874	1012	1252	1347	1529
14-17 mo	0.7695	1261.0053	0.28821	650	-159	-25	49	248	372	611	861	1000	1239	1334	1515
15-18 mo	0.7769	1251.6296	0.29074	650	-171	-36	38	238	362	602	852	991	1230	1324	1505
16-19 mo	0.7781	1244.9248	0.29231	650	-177	-42	32	231	355	595	846	984	1223	1317	1499
17-20 mo	0.7740	1240.2027	0.29311	650	-180	-46	28	227	351	590	841	979	1218	1313	1494
18-21 mo	0.7663	1235.8993	0.29350	650	-180	-47	26	224	347	586	836	975	1214	1308	1490
19-22 mo	0.7569	1229.8975	0.29388	650	-180	-49	24	220	342	580	829	968	1207	1302	1484
20-23 mo	0.7475	1220.6029	0.29460	650	-183	-53	19	213	334	571	819	957	1196	1291	1473
21-24 mo	0.7393	1206.8517	0.29591	650	-189	-61	10	202	322	557	804	941	1179	1274	1455

[a] The L, M, S values provided are estimated based on the modelling of the shifted observations (i.e. by the addition of delta to the actual increment) which explains the difference (equals to delta) in value between the "M" and the 50th centile values.

Table 8   Boys 3-month weight increments (g) - continued

Interval	L[a]	M[a]	S[a]	δ	-3SD	-2SD	-1SD	Median	+1SD	+2SD	+3SD
0-3 mo	0.6854	3638.8730	0.15801	650	1401	1899	2428	2989	3578	4194	4836
1-4 mo	0.6503	3215.1010	0.16539	650	1116	1565	2049	2565	3112	3688	4293
2-5 mo	0.5884	2661.5629	0.17708	650	758	1139	1558	2012	2500	3022	3576
3-6 mo	0.5368	2231.9042	0.18850	650	488	815	1180	1582	2021	2496	3007
4-7 mo	0.4999	1939.0717	0.19877	650	305	595	923	1289	1694	2137	2618
5-8 mo	0.4819	1745.5952	0.20848	650	179	446	751	1096	1479	1902	2365
6-9 mo	0.4866	1611.6464	0.21853	650	82	336	629	962	1334	1745	2197
7-10 mo	0.5135	1514.8958	0.22940	650	-2	248	537	865	1232	1637	2081
8-11 mo	0.5582	1442.6013	0.24108	650	-79	173	464	793	1159	1561	1998
9-12 mo	0.6092	1387.8840	0.25261	650	-148	109	405	738	1105	1506	1938
10-13 mo	0.6580	1346.3553	0.26315	650	-208	56	358	696	1066	1466	1893
11-14 mo	0.7000	1314.9304	0.27214	650	-258	13	322	665	1037	1435	1858
12-15 mo	0.7323	1291.3726	0.27922	650	-297	-20	295	641	1015	1412	1832
13-16 mo	0.7550	1273.8860	0.28446	650	-326	-44	275	624	998	1395	1811
14-17 mo	0.7695	1261.0053	0.28821	650	-346	-61	260	611	986	1382	1797
15-18 mo	0.7769	1251.6296	0.29074	650	-358	-73	250	602	977	1372	1786
16-19 mo	0.7781	1244.9248	0.29231	650	-365	-79	244	595	970	1366	1779
17-20 mo	0.7740	1240.2027	0.29311	650	-366	-82	239	590	965	1361	1775
18-21 mo	0.7663	1235.8993	0.29350	650	-365	-83	236	586	960	1357	1772
19-22 mo	0.7569	1229.8975	0.29388	650	-363	-85	232	580	954	1350	1767
20-23 mo	0.7475	1220.6029	0.29460	650	-362	-89	225	571	943	1339	1756
21-24 mo	0.7393	1206.8517	0.29591	650	-365	-96	214	557	927	1322	1738

[a] The L, M, S values provided are estimated based on the modelling of the shifted observations (i.e. by the addition of delta to the actual increment) which explains the difference (equals to delta) in value between the "M" and the Median values.

Table 9   Girls 3-month weight increments (g)

Interval	L[a]	M[a]	S[a]	δ	1st	3rd	5th	15th	25th	50th	75th	85th	95th	97th	99th
0-3 mo	0.2298	3403.9240	0.16227	800	1493	1681	1784	2067	2247	2604	2992	3215	3610	3772	4089
1-4 mo	0.0924	3054.3512	0.15958	800	1293	1453	1542	1785	1941	2254	2600	2799	3159	3307	3600
2-5 mo	0.0599	2618.6440	0.16338	800	983	1120	1197	1409	1545	1819	2123	2299	2619	2751	3013
3-6 mo	0.1300	2277.5681	0.16990	800	718	843	913	1106	1229	1478	1752	1911	2197	2315	2549
4-7 mo	0.2404	2030.2917	0.17960	800	507	627	694	878	995	1230	1488	1636	1901	2009	2223
5-8 mo	0.3580	1855.0162	0.19157	800	342	461	528	710	825	1055	1305	1447	1700	1803	2005
6-9 mo	0.4576	1724.5802	0.20334	800	212	333	400	582	697	925	1170	1309	1554	1653	1846
7-10 mo	0.5317	1624.4588	0.21350	800	113	234	301	484	598	824	1066	1202	1442	1538	1724
8-11 mo	0.5891	1552.7117	0.22168	800	40	162	230	413	528	753	992	1126	1360	1454	1636
9-12 mo	0.6373	1506.4120	0.22796	800	-11	113	181	366	481	706	944	1077	1308	1401	1579
10-13 mo	0.6806	1476.5227	0.23285	800	-49	78	147	334	451	677	914	1046	1275	1366	1542
11-14 mo	0.7211	1455.9527	0.23682	800	-79	51	122	311	429	656	894	1025	1252	1342	1515
12-15 mo	0.7527	1442.0871	0.24040	800	-102	30	102	294	413	642	880	1012	1239	1328	1500
13-16 mo	0.7679	1434.2381	0.24403	800	-120	14	88	283	403	634	875	1007	1235	1325	1497
14-17 mo	0.7642	1431.1099	0.24794	800	-131	4	78	275	397	631	875	1010	1241	1333	1508
15-18 mo	0.7482	1429.1551	0.25198	800	-139	-4	70	269	392	629	877	1014	1251	1344	1524
16-19 mo	0.7267	1425.3256	0.25598	800	-147	-12	62	261	385	625	877	1017	1258	1354	1538
17-20 mo	0.7032	1418.4764	0.25989	800	-155	-21	53	252	376	618	873	1015	1261	1359	1548
18-21 mo	0.6782	1409.2288	0.26384	800	-163	-30	43	241	366	609	867	1011	1262	1361	1554
19-22 mo	0.6522	1398.1693	0.26792	800	-172	-41	32	229	354	598	859	1005	1260	1362	1559
20-23 mo	0.6262	1385.3711	0.27191	800	-181	-52	20	216	340	585	848	996	1255	1359	1560
21-24 mo	0.6013	1370.5464	0.27539	800	-190	-63	8	202	326	571	834	984	1246	1351	1556

[a] The L, M, S values provided are estimated based on the modelling of the shifted observations (i.e. by the addition of delta to the actual increment) which explains the difference (equals to delta) in value between the "M" and the 50th centile values.

Table 9 Girls 3-month weight increments (g) - continued

Interval	L[a]	M[a]	S[a]	δ	-3SD	-2SD	-1SD	Median	+1SD	+2SD	+3SD
0-3 mo	0.2298	3403.9240	0.16227	800	1231	1629	2085	2604	3192	3855	4600
1-4 mo	0.0924	3054.3512	0.15958	800	1072	1409	1801	2254	2779	3383	4079
2-5 mo	0.0599	2618.6440	0.16338	800	792	1083	1422	1819	2281	2819	3445
3-6 mo	0.1300	2277.5681	0.16990	800	544	809	1118	1478	1894	2376	2931
4-7 mo	0.2404	2030.2917	0.17960	800	340	594	890	1230	1621	2065	2570
5-8 mo	0.3580	1855.0162	0.19157	800	175	429	721	1055	1433	1856	2328
6-9 mo	0.4576	1724.5802	0.20334	800	43	300	593	925	1295	1704	2153
7-10 mo	0.5317	1624.4588	0.21350	800	-58	201	495	824	1189	1587	2019
8-11 mo	0.5891	1552.7117	0.22168	800	-132	129	424	753	1112	1502	1921
9-12 mo	0.6373	1506.4120	0.22796	800	-186	79	378	706	1064	1448	1857
10-13 mo	0.6806	1476.5227	0.23285	800	-228	43	346	677	1033	1413	1815
11-14 mo	0.7211	1455.9527	0.23682	800	-262	16	323	656	1012	1388	1784
12-15 mo	0.7527	1442.0871	0.24040	800	-290	-6	306	642	999	1374	1766
13-16 mo	0.7679	1434.2381	0.24403	800	-311	-22	295	634	994	1371	1764
14-17 mo	0.7642	1431.1099	0.24794	800	-323	-33	287	631	996	1379	1779
15-18 mo	0.7482	1429.1551	0.25198	800	-331	-41	281	629	1000	1392	1802
16-19 mo	0.7267	1425.3256	0.25598	800	-337	-49	274	625	1002	1403	1824
17-20 mo	0.7032	1418.4764	0.25989	800	-342	-57	265	618	1001	1409	1841
18-21 mo	0.6782	1409.2288	0.26384	800	-347	-67	254	609	996	1412	1856
19-22 mo	0.6522	1398.1693	0.26792	800	-352	-77	242	598	990	1414	1868
20-23 mo	0.6262	1385.3711	0.27191	800	-358	-87	228	585	981	1412	1878
21-24 mo	0.6013	1370.5464	0.27539	800	-363	-98	214	571	968	1406	1880

[a] The L, M, S values provided are estimated based on the modelling of the shifted observations (i.e. by the addition of delta to the actual increment) which explains the difference (equals to delta) in value between the "M" and the Median values.

Table 10 Boys 4-month weight increments (g)

Interval	L[a]	M[a]	S[a]	δ	1st	3rd	5th	15th	25th	50th	75th	85th	95th	97th	99th
0-4 mo	0.7672	4136.2992	0.15684	500	2196	2460	2603	2977	3204	3636	4079	4321	4734	4896	5206
1-5 mo	0.6482	3623.4564	0.17439	500	1763	2006	2138	2490	2706	3123	3558	3799	4214	4378	4695
2-6 mo	0.5632	2900.4470	0.19057	500	1242	1444	1554	1852	2038	2400	2784	2998	3371	3520	3809
3-7 mo	0.4863	2424.1094	0.20390	500	914	1086	1181	1440	1602	1924	2269	2464	2807	2946	3215
4-8 mo	0.4302	2106.5547	0.21598	500	696	848	933	1165	1312	1607	1926	2108	2432	2563	2820
5-9 mo	0.4321	1871.4914	0.22766	500	526	666	744	959	1097	1371	1671	1843	2148	2272	2515
6-10 mo	0.4881	1711.6071	0.24076	500	390	526	602	812	945	1212	1501	1666	1958	2077	2308
7-11 mo	0.5825	1598.0178	0.25575	500	270	409	486	698	832	1098	1384	1545	1828	1942	2163
8-12 mo	0.6678	1526.3463	0.27024	500	175	320	401	619	757	1026	1313	1473	1753	1864	2080
9-13 mo	0.7242	1473.6287	0.28350	500	101	251	334	559	700	974	1263	1423	1702	1813	2027
10-14 mo	0.7587	1423.7181	0.29393	500	43	195	280	507	648	924	1213	1373	1649	1759	1970
11-15 mo	0.7822	1370.5468	0.30204	500	-6	147	231	457	598	871	1156	1313	1585	1693	1899
12-16 mo	0.7966	1334.9524	0.30757	500	-37	115	199	424	564	835	1118	1274	1542	1648	1852
13-17 mo	0.8054	1321.4376	0.31114	500	-54	99	183	410	550	821	1104	1260	1528	1634	1837
14-18 mo	0.8084	1315.2621	0.31327	500	-62	91	175	403	543	815	1099	1255	1523	1630	1833
15-19 mo	0.8041	1308.5472	0.31429	500	-66	87	171	397	537	809	1091	1248	1516	1622	1826
16-20 mo	0.7912	1297.8646	0.31482	500	-66	84	167	390	529	798	1079	1235	1503	1609	1813
17-21 mo	0.7712	1284.7539	0.31520	500	-64	82	163	382	519	785	1064	1219	1487	1593	1797
18-22 mo	0.7469	1271.4590	0.31566	500	-62	80	159	374	508	771	1049	1204	1472	1578	1783
19-23 mo	0.7222	1262.1643	0.31628	500	-58	80	157	368	501	762	1039	1194	1463	1570	1777
20-24 mo	0.6991	1257.3339	0.31696	500	-54	81	157	366	497	757	1035	1190	1461	1570	1779

[a] The L, M, S values provided are estimated based on the modelling of the shifted observations (i.e. by the addition of delta to the actual increment) which explains the difference (equals to delta) in value between the "M" and the 50th centile values.

Table 10   Boys 4-month weight increments (g) - *continued*

Interval	L[a]	M[a]	S[a]	δ	-3SD	-2SD	-1SD	Median	+1SD	+2SD	+3SD
0-4 mo	0.7672	4136.2992	0.15684	500	1807	2389	3000	3636	4297	4979	5681
1-5 mo	0.6482	3623.4564	0.17439	500	1413	1940	2511	3123	3774	4462	5186
2-6 mo	0.5632	2900.4470	0.19057	500	955	1389	1871	2400	2976	3597	4261
3-7 mo	0.4863	2424.1094	0.20390	500	673	1039	1456	1924	2444	3017	3641
4-8 mo	0.4302	2106.5547	0.21598	500	486	806	1179	1607	2090	2631	3231
5-9 mo	0.4321	1871.4914	0.22766	500	333	627	973	1371	1825	2336	2905
6-10 mo	0.4881	1711.6071	0.24076	500	202	489	825	1212	1649	2138	2678
7-11 mo	0.5825	1598.0178	0.25575	500	78	371	711	1098	1528	2000	2513
8-12 mo	0.6678	1526.3463	0.27024	500	-25	281	633	1026	1457	1921	2418
9-13 mo	0.7242	1473.6287	0.28350	500	-107	210	573	974	1407	1870	2359
10-14 mo	0.7587	1423.7181	0.29393	500	-168	154	521	924	1356	1815	2297
11-15 mo	0.7822	1370.5468	0.30204	500	-217	105	471	871	1297	1748	2219
12-16 mo	0.7966	1334.9524	0.30757	500	-248	73	438	835	1258	1702	2166
13-17 mo	0.8054	1321.4376	0.31114	500	-266	57	424	821	1244	1688	2151
14-18 mo	0.8084	1315.2621	0.31327	500	-275	49	416	815	1239	1684	2146
15-19 mo	0.8041	1308.5472	0.31429	500	-276	45	411	809	1232	1676	2140
16-20 mo	0.7912	1297.8646	0.31482	500	-272	43	404	798	1219	1663	2128
17-21 mo	0.7712	1284.7539	0.31520	500	-264	42	395	785	1204	1648	2114
18-22 mo	0.7469	1271.4590	0.31566	500	-255	41	387	771	1188	1633	2102
19-23 mo	0.7222	1262.1643	0.31628	500	-245	42	381	762	1178	1625	2100
20-24 mo	0.6991	1257.3339	0.31696	500	-237	44	379	757	1174	1625	2107

[a] The L, M, S values provided are estimated based on the modelling of the shifted observations (i.e. by the addition of delta to the actual increment) which explains the difference (equals to delta) in value between the "M" and the Median values.

Table 11 Girls 4-month weight increments (g)

Interval	L[a]	M[a]	S[a]	δ	1st	3rd	5th	15th	25th	50th	75th	85th	95th	97th	99th
0-4 mo	0.0891	4009.5248	0.15636	800	1970	2176	2291	2606	2806	3210	3653	3909	4370	4560	4935
1-5 mo	-0.0491	3541.1498	0.16054	800	1646	1824	1924	2200	2379	2741	3147	3385	3819	4000	4362
2-6 mo	-0.0362	3002.2985	0.16706	800	1241	1397	1484	1726	1883	2202	2561	2772	3157	3318	3641
3-7 mo	0.0557	2616.8194	0.17682	800	926	1071	1152	1377	1522	1817	2147	2340	2692	2838	3130
4-8 mo	0.1899	2331.5089	0.18968	800	671	811	890	1108	1248	1532	1846	2028	2357	2493	2762
5-9 mo	0.3154	2118.7222	0.20292	800	471	611	689	904	1042	1319	1623	1797	2110	2238	2490
6-10 mo	0.4069	1963.5334	0.21481	800	323	463	541	755	891	1164	1460	1630	1932	2054	2295
7-11 mo	0.4873	1855.0205	0.22441	800	216	356	435	649	785	1055	1347	1512	1805	1923	2154
8-12 mo	0.5659	1780.1251	0.23120	800	137	281	360	576	712	980	1267	1429	1712	1826	2047
9-13 mo	0.6483	1726.3407	0.23622	800	75	222	303	522	659	926	1209	1367	1641	1751	1962
10-14 mo	0.7201	1691.6549	0.23980	800	29	181	264	486	624	892	1171	1326	1594	1700	1904
11-15 mo	0.7759	1668.6291	0.24275	800	-6	150	235	461	601	869	1147	1300	1563	1667	1865
12-16 mo	0.8064	1655.3840	0.24522	800	-29	130	216	446	586	855	1133	1286	1547	1650	1847
13-17 mo	0.8111	1648.5922	0.24757	800	-41	119	206	436	578	849	1128	1281	1544	1647	1845
14-18 mo	0.7924	1643.8520	0.25015	800	-47	112	199	430	572	844	1126	1281	1547	1652	1853
15-19 mo	0.7577	1638.7127	0.25299	800	-48	108	194	423	565	839	1124	1281	1553	1660	1866
16-20 mo	0.7139	1631.2189	0.25623	800	-50	104	188	415	556	831	1120	1280	1558	1668	1880
17-21 mo	0.6699	1621.0212	0.25952	800	-52	98	180	405	546	821	1113	1276	1560	1673	1891
18-22 mo	0.6227	1607.4454	0.26290	800	-56	90	171	392	532	807	1102	1267	1557	1674	1899
19-23 mo	0.5732	1591.7399	0.26613	800	-59	82	162	379	517	792	1088	1256	1552	1672	1904
20-24 mo	0.5249	1576.2729	0.26914	800	-62	75	152	366	503	776	1075	1245	1547	1669	1909

[a] The L, M, S values provided are estimated based on the modelling of the shifted observations (i.e. by the addition of delta to the actual increment) which explains the difference (equals to delta) in value between the "M" and the 50th centile values.

Table 11 Girls 4-month weight increments (g) - continued

Interval	L[a]	M[a]	S[a]	δ	-3SD	-2SD	-1SD	Median	+1SD	+2SD	+3SD
0-4 mo	0.0891	4009.5248	0.15636	800	1683	2120	2625	3210	3883	4658	5548
1-5 mo	-0.0491	3541.1498	0.16054	800	1400	1775	2218	2741	3360	4094	4965
2-6 mo	-0.0362	3002.2985	0.16706	800	1027	1354	1742	2202	2750	3402	4179
3-7 mo	0.0557	2616.8194	0.17682	800	727	1031	1391	1817	2320	2914	3614
4-8 mo	0.1899	2331.5089	0.18968	800	477	773	1122	1532	2009	2563	3202
5-9 mo	0.3154	2118.7222	0.20292	800	278	572	918	1319	1779	2304	2898
6-10 mo	0.4069	1963.5334	0.21481	800	130	424	768	1164	1613	2117	2680
7-11 mo	0.4873	1855.0205	0.22441	800	20	318	663	1055	1495	1984	2521
8-12 mo	0.5659	1780.1251	0.23120	800	-62	241	589	980	1412	1884	2396
9-13 mo	0.6483	1726.3407	0.23622	800	-132	182	536	926	1351	1807	2293
10-14 mo	0.7201	1691.6549	0.23980	800	-186	139	500	892	1310	1754	2220
11-15 mo	0.7759	1668.6291	0.24275	800	-229	107	475	869	1284	1719	2172
12-16 mo	0.8064	1655.3840	0.24522	800	-257	87	460	855	1271	1702	2149
13-17 mo	0.8111	1648.5922	0.24757	800	-271	75	451	849	1266	1700	2148
14-18 mo	0.7924	1643.8520	0.25015	800	-274	69	444	844	1265	1705	2162
15-19 mo	0.7577	1638.7127	0.25299	800	-270	66	437	839	1265	1715	2185
16-20 mo	0.7139	1631.2189	0.25623	800	-265	62	429	831	1264	1725	2210
17-21 mo	0.6699	1621.0212	0.25952	800	-261	57	419	821	1259	1731	2233
18-22 mo	0.6227	1607.4454	0.26290	800	-257	50	406	807	1251	1733	2253
19-23 mo	0.5732	1591.7399	0.26613	800	-253	44	393	792	1239	1733	2272
20-24 mo	0.5249	1576.2729	0.26914	800	-249	37	379	776	1228	1732	2290

[a] The L, M, S values provided are estimated based on the modelling of the shifted observations (i.e. by the addition of delta to the actual increment) which explains the difference (equals to delta) in value between the "M" and the Median values.

Table 12   Boys 6-month weight increments (g)

Interval	L[a]	M[a]	S[a]	δ	1st	3rd	5th	15th	25th	50th	75th	85th	95th	97th	99th
0-6 mo	0.5209	4929.7718	0.15679	350	2940	3229	3387	3810	4072	4580	5114	5412	5929	6136	6534
1-7 mo	0.4856	4243.2925	0.17552	350	2342	2611	2759	3157	3406	3893	4411	4701	5210	5413	5809
2-8 mo	0.4609	3442.9150	0.19228	350	1736	1968	2096	2443	2662	3093	3555	3816	4275	4461	4821
3-9 mo	0.4490	2879.5905	0.20802	350	1319	1523	1636	1945	2141	2530	2949	3188	3609	3779	4112
4-10 mo	0.4511	2501.8054	0.22426	350	1030	1217	1321	1607	1789	2152	2546	2771	3169	3331	3647
5-11 mo	0.4660	2220.6833	0.24197	350	806	982	1080	1351	1524	1871	2249	2465	2849	3005	3311
6-12 mo	0.4895	2037.9406	0.26076	350	642	813	909	1175	1346	1688	2062	2277	2658	2813	3116
7-13 mo	0.5168	1903.1830	0.27848	350	515	683	778	1042	1212	1553	1927	2141	2521	2675	2978
8-14 mo	0.5442	1794.7774	0.29319	350	415	582	676	938	1106	1445	1816	2028	2404	2557	2856
9-15 mo	0.5697	1709.1588	0.30394	350	341	506	599	858	1024	1359	1725	1934	2304	2453	2746
10-16 mo	0.5943	1651.4150	0.31109	350	291	455	547	805	970	1301	1662	1868	2232	2379	2665
11-17 mo	0.6190	1616.6162	0.31517	350	258	422	515	772	937	1267	1624	1827	2184	2329	2609
12-18 mo	0.6428	1590.6081	0.31683	350	236	400	493	750	914	1241	1593	1793	2143	2284	2558
13-19 mo	0.6649	1571.5549	0.31675	350	221	386	479	735	898	1222	1569	1765	2108	2246	2513
14-20 mo	0.6849	1557.0267	0.31549	350	212	377	470	725	887	1207	1549	1741	2077	2212	2472
15-21 mo	0.7027	1545.9058	0.31347	350	206	372	465	719	880	1196	1533	1721	2050	2182	2435
16-22 mo	0.7187	1533.6871	0.31113	350	202	368	460	713	872	1184	1515	1700	2021	2150	2397
17-23 mo	0.7336	1520.6160	0.30878	350	198	363	455	706	863	1171	1496	1677	1992	2117	2358
18-24 mo	0.7478	1508.4744	0.30647	350	195	360	451	700	855	1158	1478	1656	1964	2086	2321

[a] The L, M, S values provided are estimated based on the modelling of the shifted observations (i.e. by the addition of delta to the actual increment) which explains the difference (equals to delta) in value between the "M" and the 50th centile values.

Table 12 Boys 6-month weight increments (g) – *continued*

Interval	L[a]	M[a]	S[a]	δ	-3SD	-2SD	-1SD	Median	+1SD	+2SD	+3SD
0-6 mo	0.5209	4929.7718	0.15679	350	2524	3151	3836	4580	5382	6241	7158
1-7 mo	0.4856	4243.2925	0.17552	350	1960	2538	3182	3893	4672	5518	6432
2-8 mo	0.4609	3442.9150	0.19228	350	1411	1905	2465	3093	3789	4556	5392
3-9 mo	0.4490	2879.5905	0.20802	350	1035	1467	1965	2530	3163	3867	4642
4-10 mo	0.4511	2501.8054	0.22426	350	772	1166	1625	2152	2748	3414	4152
5-11 mo	0.4660	2220.6833	0.24197	350	566	933	1368	1871	2443	3086	3800
6-12 mo	0.4895	2037.9406	0.26076	350	410	766	1192	1688	2255	2893	3602
7-13 mo	0.5168	1903.1830	0.27848	350	288	637	1059	1553	2119	2755	3461
8-14 mo	0.5442	1794.7774	0.29319	350	192	536	954	1445	2006	2636	3333
9-15 mo	0.5697	1709.1588	0.30394	350	122	460	874	1359	1912	2531	3212
10-16 mo	0.5943	1651.4150	0.31109	350	73	409	821	1301	1847	2454	3120
11-17 mo	0.6190	1616.6162	0.31517	350	40	377	789	1267	1806	2403	3053
12-18 mo	0.6428	1590.6081	0.31683	350	16	355	766	1241	1772	2357	2990
13-19 mo	0.6649	1571.5549	0.31675	350	0	340	751	1222	1745	2316	2932
14-20 mo	0.6849	1557.0267	0.31549	350	-11	331	741	1207	1722	2281	2880
15-21 mo	0.7027	1545.9058	0.31347	350	-18	326	735	1196	1702	2249	2832
16-22 mo	0.7187	1533.6871	0.31113	350	-23	322	728	1184	1681	2215	2783
17-23 mo	0.7336	1520.6160	0.30878	350	-27	318	721	1171	1659	2181	2733
18-24 mo	0.7478	1508.4744	0.30647	350	-31	314	715	1158	1638	2148	2687

[a] The L, M, S values provided are estimated based on the modelling of the shifted observations (i.e. by the addition of delta to the actual increment) which explains the difference (equals to delta) in value between the "M" and the Median values.

Table 13 Girls 6-month weight increments (g)

Interval	L[a]	M[a]	S[a]	δ	1st	3rd	5th	15th	25th	50th	75th	85th	95th	97th	99th
0-6 mo	-0.1223	4528.9831	0.15945	450	2701	2924	3049	3395	3620	4079	4597	4902	5462	5697	6170
1-7 mo	-0.0280	3911.9319	0.17265	450	2174	2381	2498	2822	3033	3462	3946	4231	4753	4971	5409
2-8 mo	0.0799	3327.7315	0.18755	450	1684	1877	1985	2286	2480	2878	3324	3586	4063	4262	4660
3-9 mo	0.1942	2853.3800	0.20514	450	1279	1461	1563	1846	2030	2403	2821	3064	3506	3689	4054
4-10 mo	0.3097	2501.5063	0.22466	450	964	1140	1240	1514	1692	2052	2451	2682	3099	3271	3610
5-11 mo	0.4246	2248.5880	0.24383	450	725	900	999	1271	1446	1799	2186	2409	2807	2969	3288
6-12 mo	0.5250	2068.2742	0.25997	450	549	725	824	1097	1271	1618	1996	2211	2592	2746	3047
7-13 mo	0.6042	1939.2944	0.27156	450	425	603	702	975	1147	1489	1857	2065	2430	2577	2862
8-14 mo	0.6644	1850.4715	0.27943	450	340	519	619	891	1063	1400	1760	1962	2314	2454	2726
9-15 mo	0.7065	1793.3361	0.28481	450	284	465	565	838	1009	1343	1697	1895	2238	2375	2638
10-16 mo	0.7288	1758.5512	0.28870	450	249	431	532	805	975	1309	1660	1855	2194	2329	2588
11-17 mo	0.7317	1738.3567	0.29175	450	230	412	513	785	956	1288	1639	1834	2173	2307	2566
12-18 mo	0.7206	1725.0429	0.29439	450	221	401	501	772	942	1275	1627	1823	2163	2299	2560
13-19 mo	0.7016	1713.8691	0.29696	450	216	394	492	762	931	1264	1617	1815	2158	2296	2560
14-20 mo	0.6812	1703.1167	0.29971	450	211	386	484	751	920	1253	1608	1807	2155	2294	2563
15-21 mo	0.6643	1691.6943	0.30278	450	204	377	474	740	908	1242	1599	1800	2151	2292	2565
16-22 mo	0.6534	1677.6772	0.30619	450	193	365	461	726	894	1228	1586	1788	2143	2285	2561
17-23 mo	0.6489	1659.9660	0.30991	450	178	348	444	708	876	1210	1569	1772	2128	2271	2549
18-24 mo	0.6476	1640.7438	0.31376	450	161	330	425	689	857	1191	1551	1754	2111	2254	2533

[a] The L, M, S values provided are estimated based on the modelling of the shifted observations (i.e. by the addition of delta to the actual increment) which explains the difference (equals to delta) in value between the "M" and the 50th centile values.

Table 13 Girls 6-month weight increments (g) - continued

Interval	L[a]	M[a]	S[a]	δ	-3SD	-2SD	-1SD	Median	+1SD	+2SD	+3SD
0-6 mo	-0.1223	4528.9831	0.15945	450	2395	2862	3417	4079	4870	5820	6964
1-7 mo	-0.0280	3911.9319	0.17265	450	1889	2324	2843	3462	4201	5085	6141
2-8 mo	0.0799	3327.7315	0.18755	450	1421	1824	2305	2878	3559	4366	5320
3-9 mo	0.1942	2853.3800	0.20514	450	1032	1411	1864	2403	3039	3784	4653
4-10 mo	0.3097	2501.5063	0.22466	450	725	1092	1532	2052	2658	3360	4164
5-11 mo	0.4246	2248.5880	0.24383	450	486	852	1288	1799	2386	3053	3802
6-12 mo	0.5250	2068.2742	0.25997	450	308	677	1114	1618	2189	2825	3527
7-13 mo	0.6042	1939.2944	0.27156	450	182	554	992	1489	2044	2652	3311
8-14 mo	0.6644	1850.4715	0.27943	450	93	470	908	1400	1941	2526	3153
9-15 mo	0.7065	1793.3361	0.28481	450	34	415	855	1343	1875	2444	3049
10-16 mo	0.7288	1758.5512	0.28870	450	-2	381	822	1309	1835	2397	2991
11-17 mo	0.7317	1738.3567	0.29175	450	-20	362	802	1288	1815	2376	2969
12-18 mo	0.7206	1725.0429	0.29439	450	-26	352	789	1275	1803	2368	2967
13-19 mo	0.7016	1713.8691	0.29696	450	-27	345	778	1264	1795	2366	2974
14-20 mo	0.6812	1703.1167	0.29971	450	-26	338	768	1253	1787	2365	2984
15-21 mo	0.6643	1691.6943	0.30278	450	-30	330	756	1242	1779	2364	2993
16-22 mo	0.6534	1677.6772	0.30619	450	-38	317	742	1228	1768	2358	2995
17-23 mo	0.6489	1659.9660	0.30991	450	-51	301	724	1210	1752	2345	2986
18-24 mo	0.6476	1640.7438	0.31376	450	-66	283	705	1191	1733	2328	2972

[a] The L, M, S values provided are estimated based on the modelling of the shifted observations (i.e. by the addition of delta to the actual increment) which explains the difference (equals to delta) in value between the "M" and the Median values.

Appendix A3 Diagnostics

A3.1a 1-month intervals for boys

Table A3.1   Q-test for z-scores from selected model [BCPE(x=age$^{0.05}$, df(μ)=9, df(σ)=4, df(v)=4, τ=2)] for 1-month weight velocity for boys

Age (days)	Group	N	z1	z2	z3
26 to 44	**0-1 mo**	419	-0.4	0.7	-0.1
44 to 76	**1-2 mo**	417	0.9	-0.3	1.4
76 to 107	**2-3 mo**	415	-0.6	-0.5	0.4
107 to 137	**3-4 mo**	405	0.0	-0.5	-0.3
137 to 168	**4-5 mo**	406	1.0	-1.5	0.2
168 to 198	**5-6 mo**	408	-0.9	1.8	-0.6
198 to 229	**6-7 mo**	410	-0.2	0.4	-1.0
229 to 259	**7-8 mo**	406	0.0	0.2	2.2
259 to 289	**8-9 mo**	396	0.4	-0.3	0.1
289 to 320	**9-10 mo**	392	0.1	-0.8	0.0
320 to 350	**10-11 mo**	396	-0.8	0.5	-0.2
350 to 370	**11-12 mo**	399	0.4	0.3	0.0
Overall Q stats		4869	4.3	7.8	8.3
degrees of freedom			3.0	9.5	8.0
p-value			0.2272	0.5994	0.4060

Note: Absolute values of z1, z2 or z3 larger than 2 indicate misfit of, respectively, mean, variance or skewness.

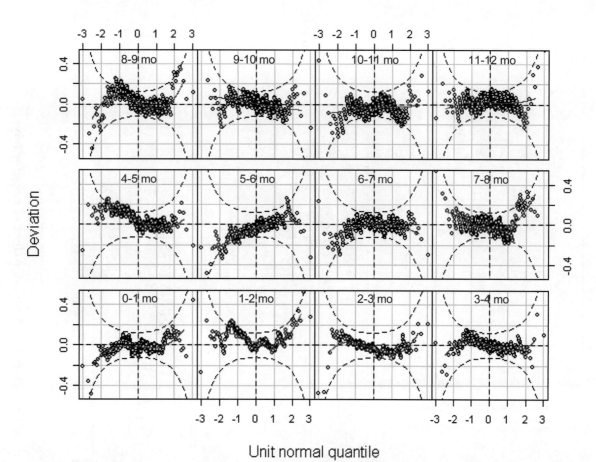

Figure A3.1 Worm plots from selected model [BCPE(x=age$^{0.05}$, df(μ)=9, df(σ)=4, df(ν)=4, τ=2)] for 1-month weight velocity for boys

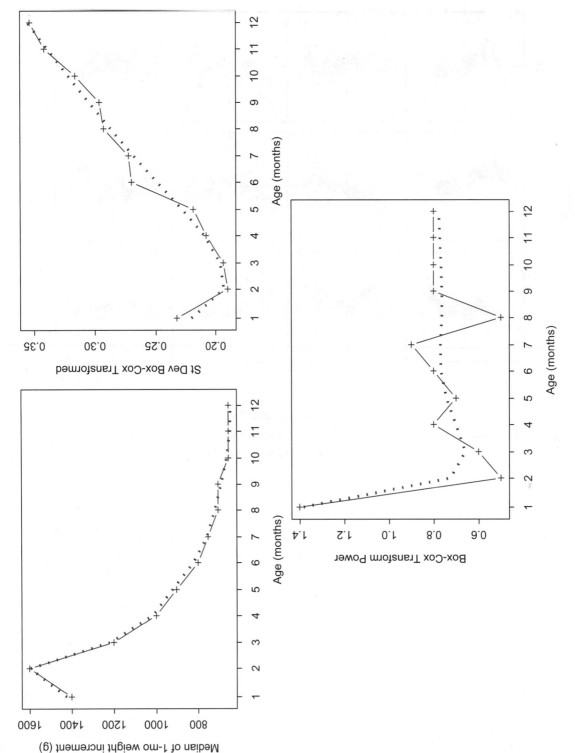

Figure A3.2 Fitting of the μ, σ, and ν curves of selected model for 1-month weight velocity for boys

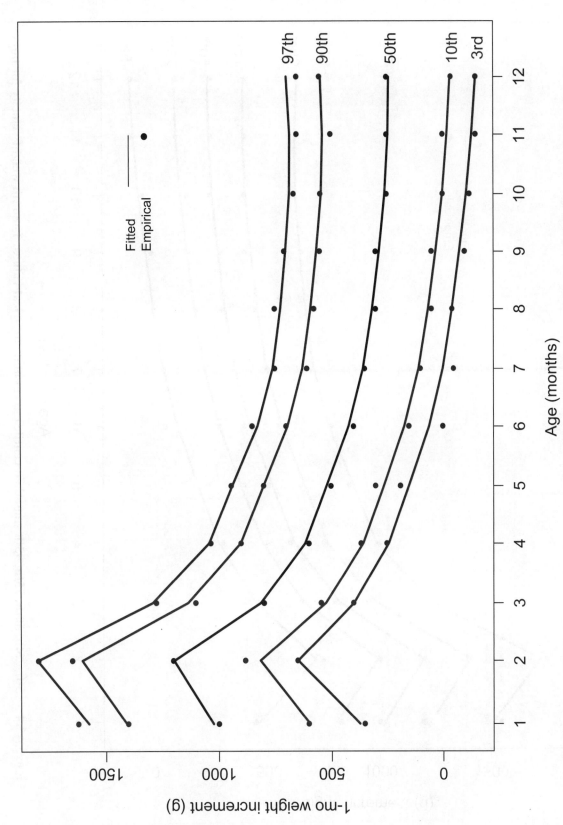

Figure A3.3   3rd, 10th, 50th, 90th, 97th smoothed centile curves and empirical values: 1-month weight velocity for boys

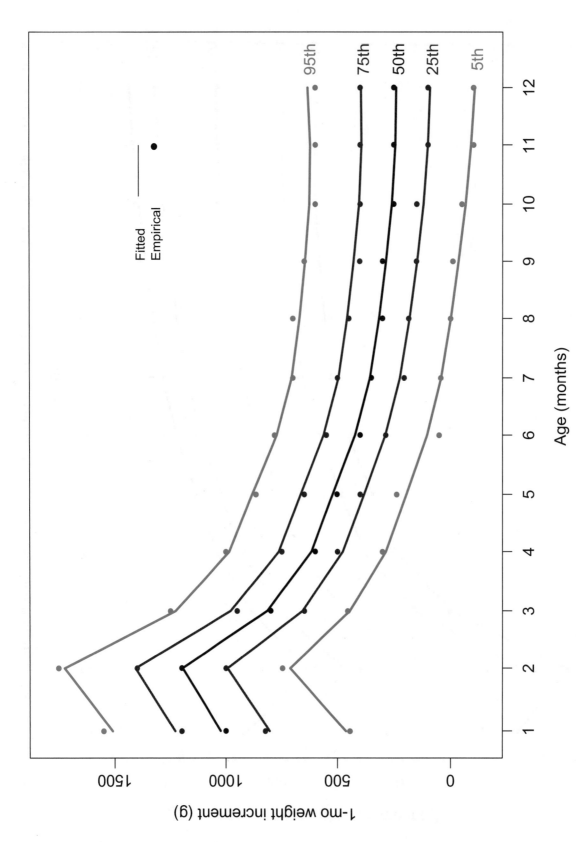

Figure A3.4   5th, 25th, 50th, 75th, 95th smoothed centile curves and empirical values: 1-month weight velocity for boys

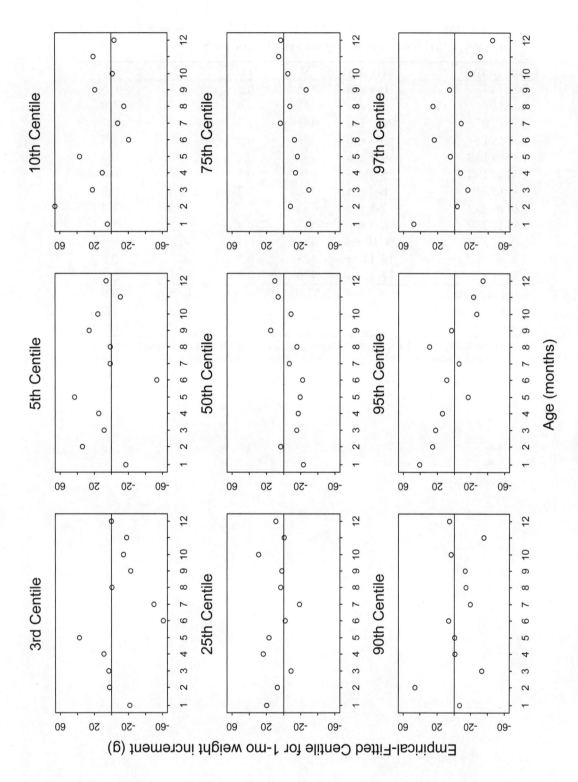

Figure A3.5 Centile residuals from fitting selected model for 1-month weight velocity for boys

A3.1b   1-month intervals for girls

Table A3.2   **Q-test for z-scores from selected model [BCPE(x=age$^{0.05}$, df(μ)=9, df(σ)=4, df(v)=1, τ=2)] for 1-month weight velocity for girls**

Age (days)	Group	N	z1	z2	z3
26 to 44	**0-1 mo**	446	-0.1	0.7	-0.5
44 to 76	**1-2 mo**	441	0.9	-0.5	1.8
76 to 107	**2-3 mo**	441	-1.0	0.5	1.7
107 to 137	**3-4 mo**	436	0.8	-2.0	-1.9
137 to 168	**4-5 mo**	438	-0.2	1.0	0.3
168 to 198	**5-6 mo**	439	0.7	-2.0	-0.6
198 to 229	**6-7 mo**	440	-1.2	1.4	-0.3
229 to 259	**7-8 mo**	433	1.1	0.5	1.4
259 to 289	**8-9 mo**	433	-0.9	1.3	-1.1
289 to 320	**9-10 mo**	431	-0.1	-0.8	1.5
320 to 350	**10-11 mo**	423	-0.1	-0.2	-0.6
350 to 370	**11-12 mo**	430	0.3	-0.1	0.4
Overall Q stats		5231	6.7	14.5	16.0
degrees of freedom			3.0	9.5	11.0
p-value			0.0832	0.1278	0.1422

Note: Absolute values of z1, z2 or z3 larger than 2 indicate misfit of, respectively, mean, variance or skewness.

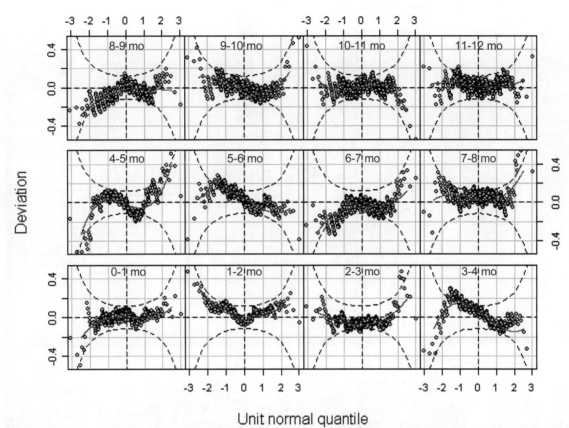

Figure A3.6 Worm plots from selected model [BCPE(x=age$^{0.05}$, df(μ)=9, df(σ)=4, df(ν)=1, τ=2)] for 1-month weight velocity for girls

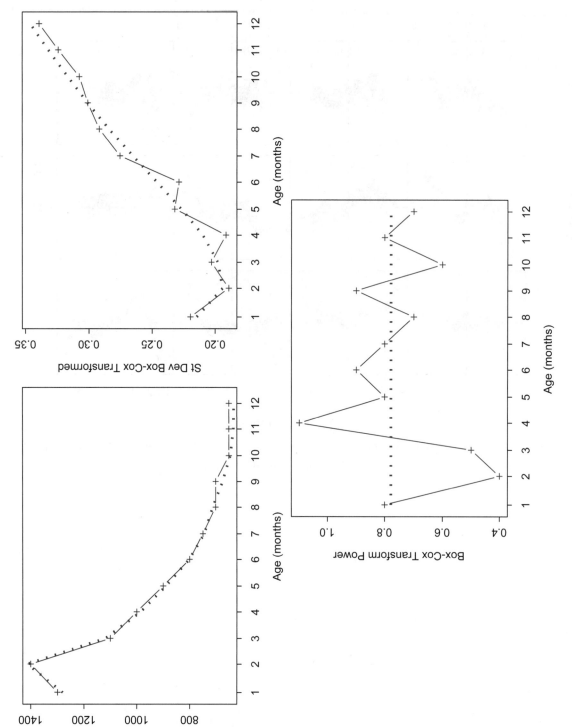

Figure A3.7 Fitting of the μ, σ, and ν curves of selected model for 1-month weight velocity for girls

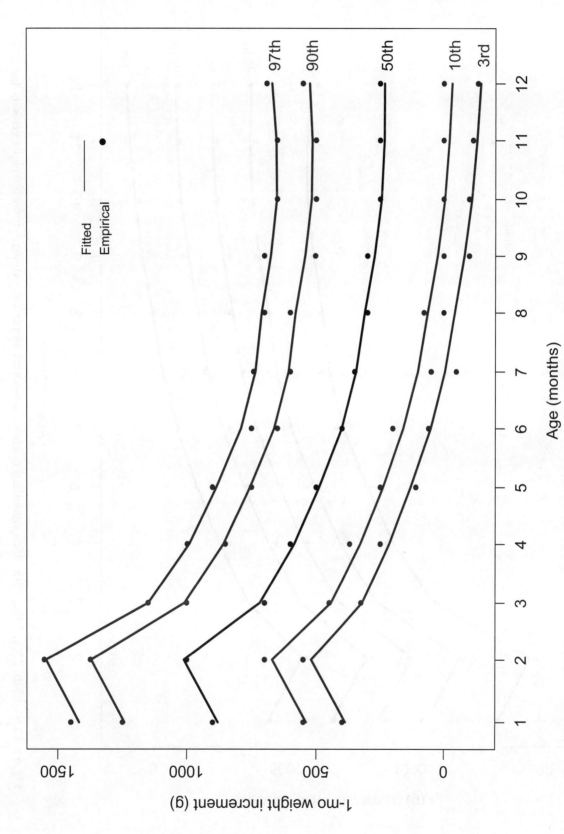

Figure A3.8 3rd, 10th, 50th, 90th, 97th smoothed centile curves and empirical values: 1-month weight velocity for girls

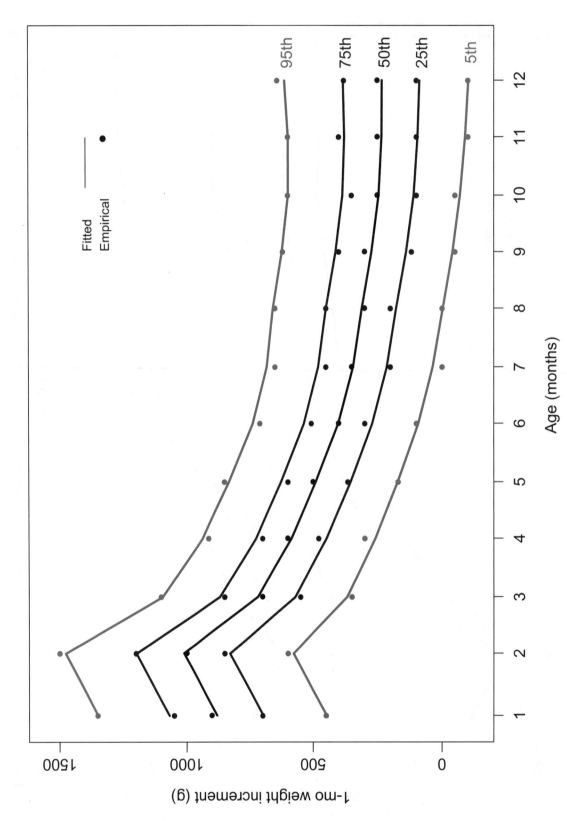

Figure A3.9   5th, 25th, 50th, 75th, 95th smoothed centile curves and empirical values: 1-month weight velocity for girls

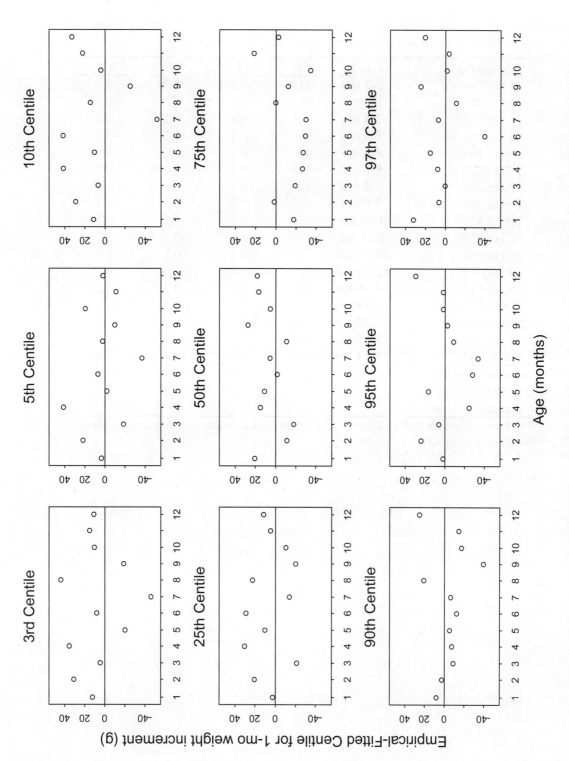

Figure A3.10 Centile residuals from fitting selected model for 1-month weight velocity for girls

A3.2a 2-month intervals for boys

Table A3.3   **Q-test for z-scores from selected model [BCPE(x=age$^{0.05}$, df(μ)=12, df(σ)=6, df(v)=3, τ=2)] for 2-month weight velocity for boys**

Age (days)	Group	N	z1	z2	z3
55 to 76	**0-2 mo**	419	-0.2	0.4	-0.7
76 to 107	**1-3 mo**	413	1.1	-0.3	-0.3
107 to 137	**2-4 mo**	407	-0.9	-0.1	1.2
137 to 168	**3-5 mo**	406	0.4	-1.1	-0.1
168 to 198	**4-6 mo**	406	0.1	1.5	-0.8
198 to 229	**5-7 mo**	404	-0.4	-0.4	0.1
229 to 259	**6-8 mo**	408	-0.1	1.0	1.9
259 to 289	**7-9 mo**	397	0.3	-0.5	1.1
289 to 320	**8-10 mo**	392	0.3	-1.3	-0.1
320 to 350	**9-11 mo**	399	-0.2	-0.8	2.3
350 to 396	**10-12 mo**	386	0.1	0.3	-1.4
396 to 457	**12-14 mo**	399	0.0	1.9	-0.2
457 to 518	**14-16 mo**	406	-1.1	0.3	-0.2
518 to 579	**16-18 mo**	406	0.8	-0.3	0.6
579 to 640	**18-20 mo**	410	-0.1	0.2	-1.4
640 to 701	**20-22 mo**	413	0.1	-0.8	1.0
701 to 738	**22-24 mo**	411	0.0	0.1	1.0
Overall Q stats		6882	4.4	11.6	19.3
degrees of freedom			5.0	13.5	14.0
p-value			0.4921	0.6004	0.1555

Note: Absolute values of z1, z2 or z3 larger than 2 indicate misfit of, respectively, mean, variance or skewness.

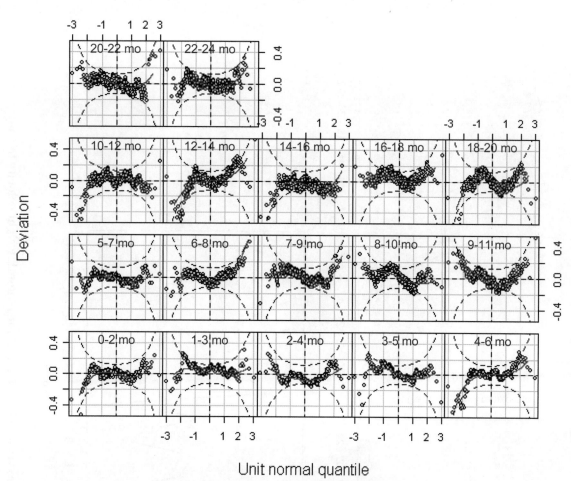

Figure A3.11 Worm plots from selected model [BCPE(x=age$^{0.05}$, df(μ)=12, df(σ)=6, df(ν)=3, τ=2)] for 2-month weight velocity for boys

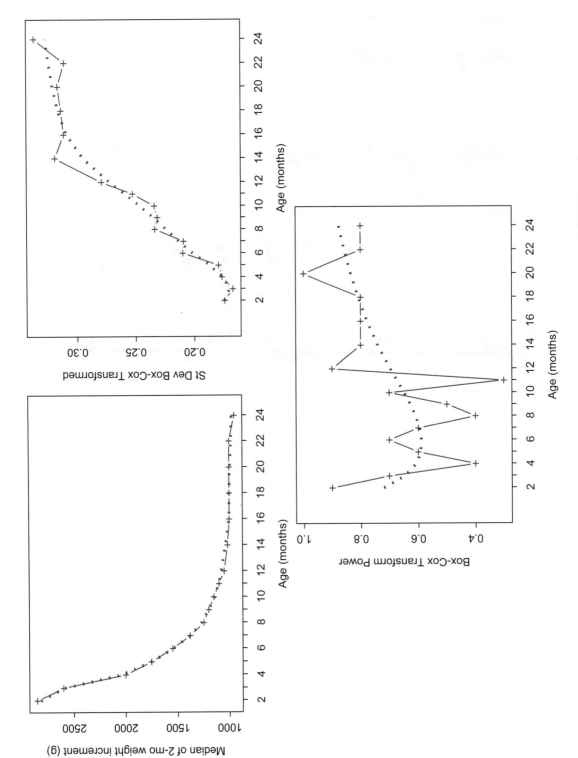

Figure A3.12 Fitting of the μ, σ, and ν curves of selected model for 2-month weight velocity for boys

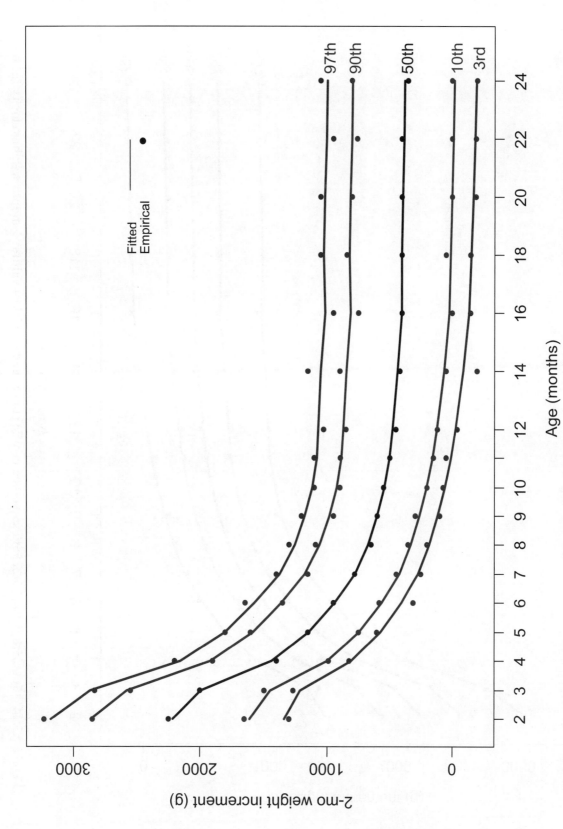

Figure A3.13   3rd, 10th, 50th, 90th, 97th smoothed centile curves and empirical values: 2-month weight velocity for boys

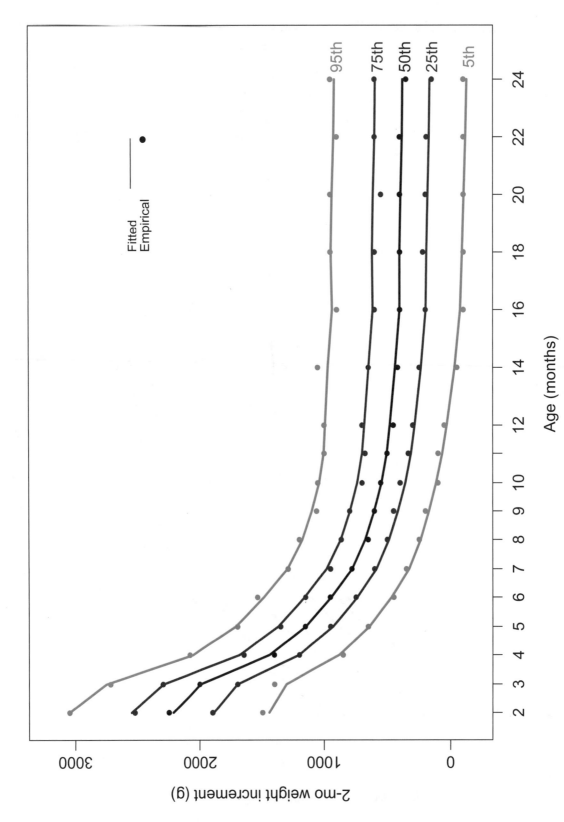

Figure A3.14   5th, 25th, 50th, 75th, 95th smoothed centile curves and empirical values; 2-month weight velocity for boys

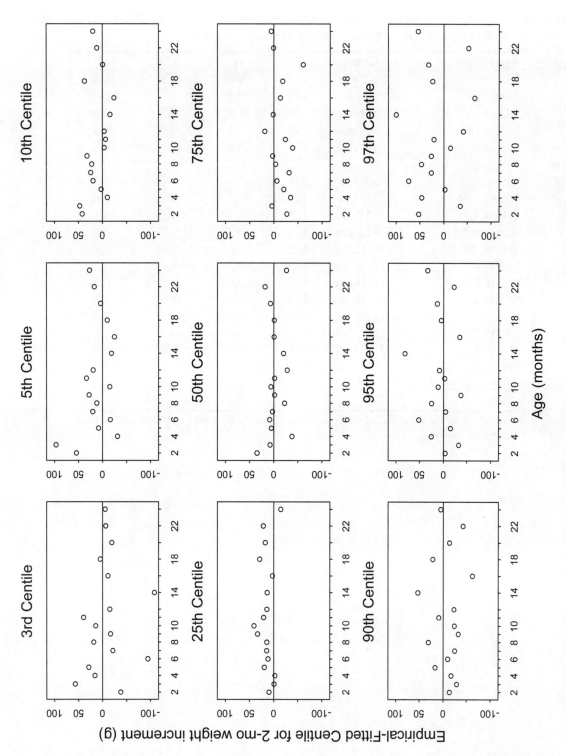

Figure A3.15 Centile residuals from fitting selected model for 2-month weight velocity for boys

A3.2b 2-month intervals for girls

Table A3.4   Q-test for z-scores from selected model   [BCPE($x=$age$^{0.05}$, df(μ)=12, df(σ)=5, df(v)=4, τ=2)] for 2-month weight velocity for girls

Age (days)	Group	N	z1	z2	z3
58 to 76	**0-2 mo**	444	0.0	0.5	-1.0
76 to 107	**1-3 mo**	440	0.5	0.2	0.9
107 to 137	**2-4 mo**	438	-0.8	-0.2	0.6
137 to 168	**3-5 mo**	440	0.4	-0.4	0.5
168 to 198	**4-6 mo**	435	0.3	-1.3	0.8
198 to 229	**5-7 mo**	437	-0.2	-1.1	-0.2
229 to 259	**6-8 mo**	435	-0.4	1.7	-0.1
259 to 289	**7-9 mo**	436	0.5	0.9	0.6
289 to 320	**8-10 mo**	425	-0.7	0.2	-0.1
320 to 350	**9-11 mo**	428	-0.3	0.6	0.4
350 to 396	**10-12 mo**	430	0.6	-1.2	1.0
396 to 457	**12-14 mo**	440	-0.2	0.7	-0.2
457 to 518	**14-16 mo**	440	-0.5	0.2	-0.4
518 to 579	**16-18 mo**	440	1.1	-1.6	-1.2
579 to 640	**18-20 mo**	437	-0.9	1.1	2.3
640 to 701	**20-22 mo**	431	1.0	-0.8	1.5
701 to 738	**22-24 mo**	433	-0.6	0.4	-0.4
Overall Q stats		7409	6.2	13.8	14.2
degrees of freedom			5.0	14.0	13.0
p-value			0.2863	0.4676	0.3632

Note: Absolute values of z1, z2 or z3 larger than 2 indicate misfit of, respectively, mean, variance or skewness.

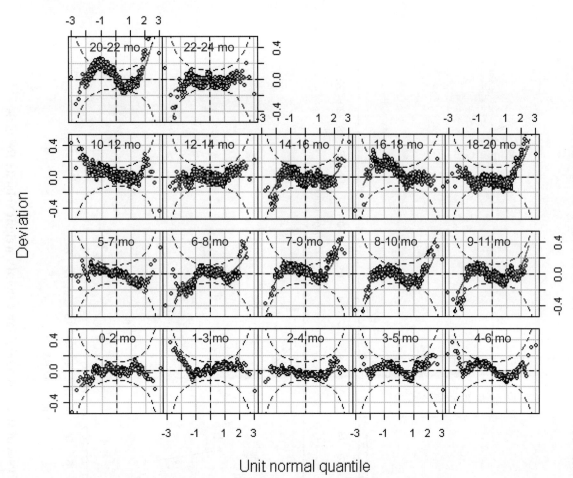

Figure A3.16 Worm plots from selected model [BCPE(x=age$^{0.05}$, df(μ)=12, df(σ)=5, df(ν)=4, τ=2)] for 2-month weight velocity for girls

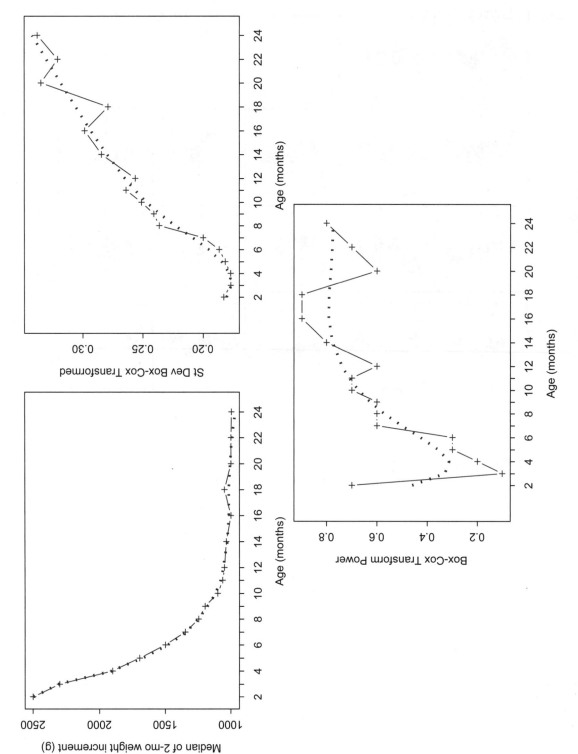

Figure A3.17 Fitting of the μ, σ, and ν curves of selected model for 2-month weight velocity for girls

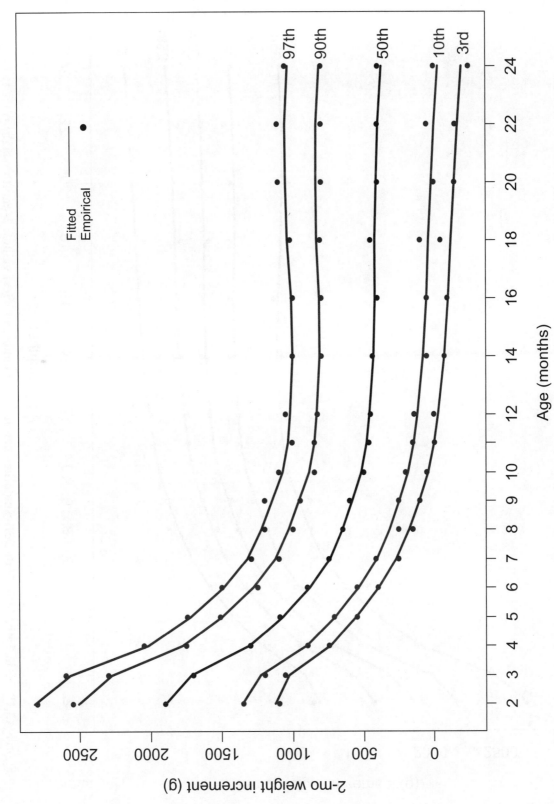

Figure A3.18   3rd, 10th, 50th, 90th, 97th smoothed centile curves and empirical values: 2-month weight velocity for girls

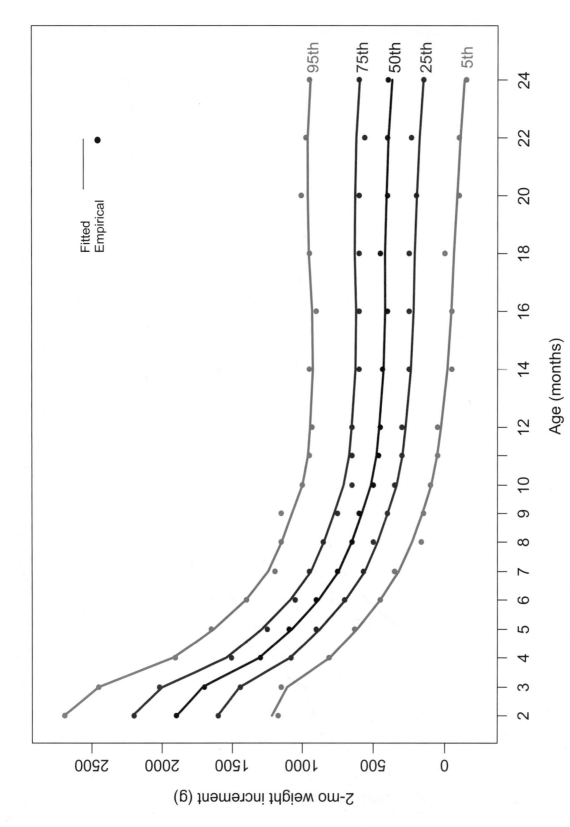

Figure A3.19 5th, 25th, 50th, 75th, 95th smoothed centile curves and empirical values: 2-month weight velocity for girls

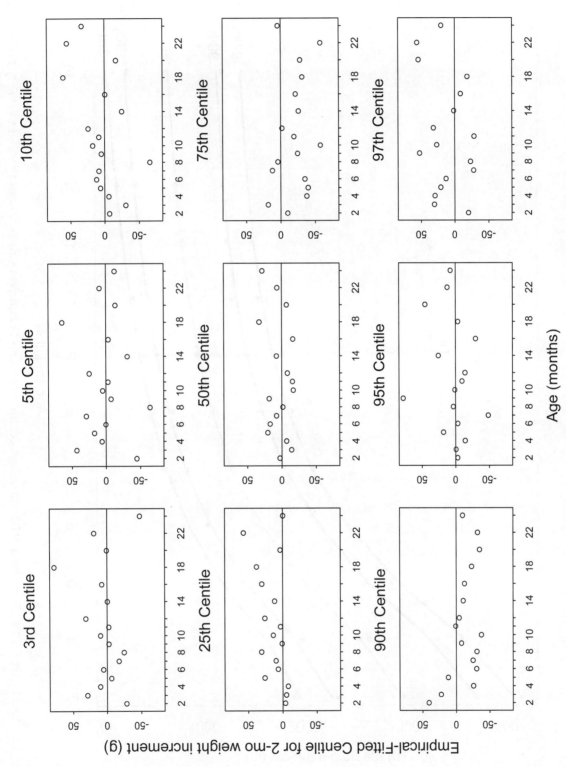

Figure A3.20 Centile residuals from fitting selected model for 2-month weight velocity for girls

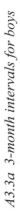

A3.3a 3-month intervals for boys

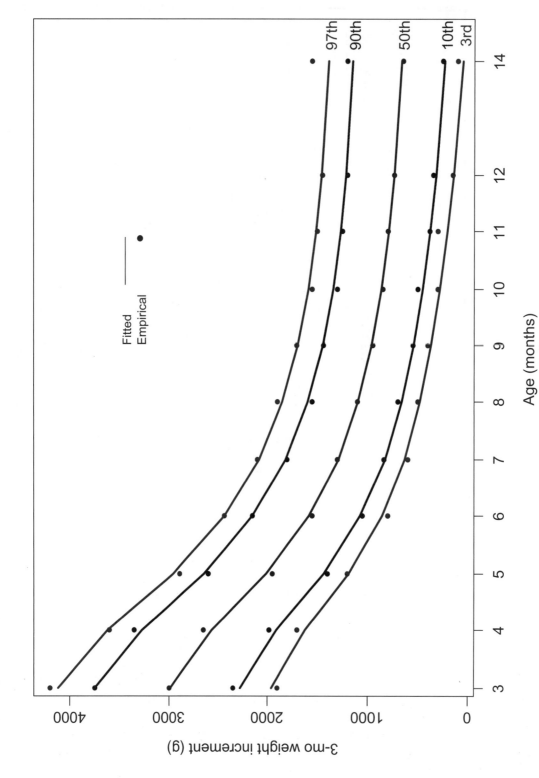

Figure A3.21 **3rd, 10th, 50th, 90th, 97th smoothed centile curves and empirical values: 3-month weight velocity for boys**

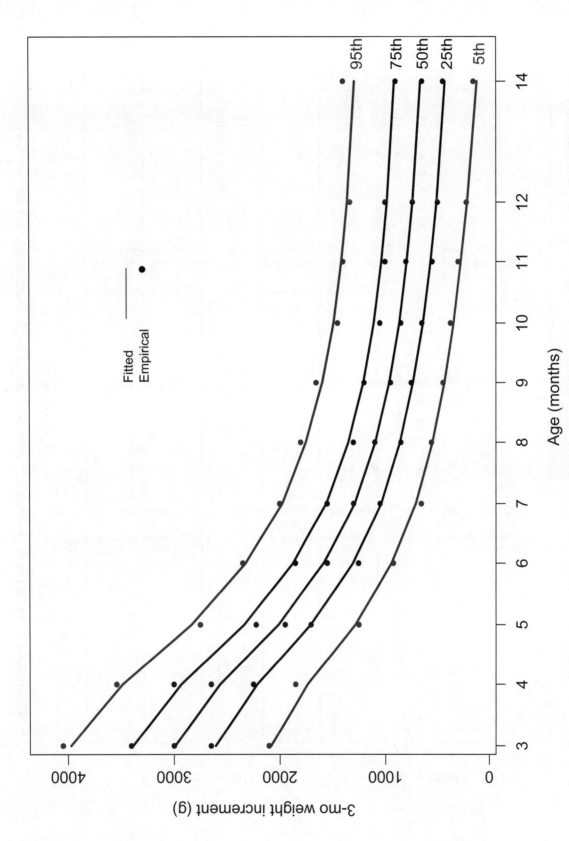

Figure A3.22 5th, 25th, 50th, 75th, 95th smoothed centile curves and empirical values: 3-month weight velocity for boys

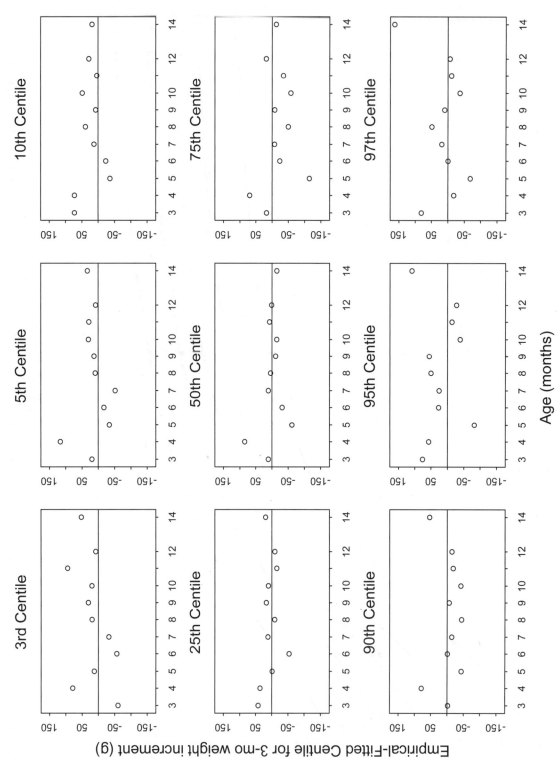

Figure A3.23 Centile residuals from fitting selected model for 3-month weight velocity for boys

A3.3b 3-month intervals for girls

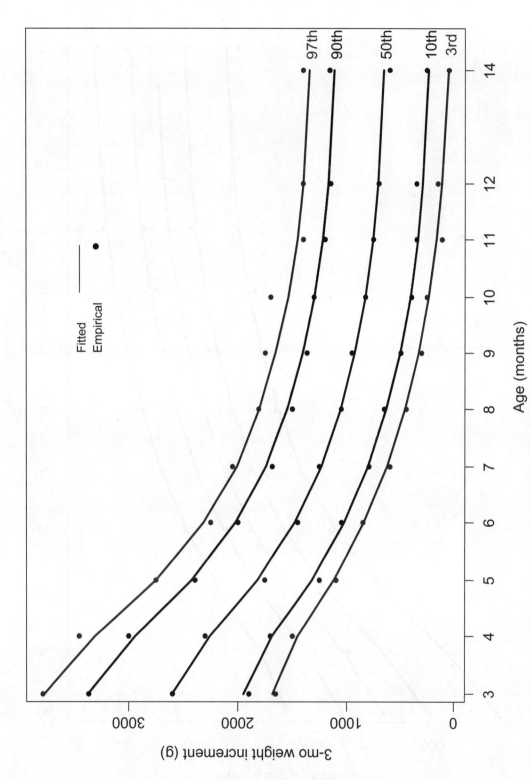

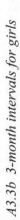

Figure A3.24   3rd, 10th, 50th, 90th, 97th smoothed centile curves and empirical values: 3-month weight velocity for girls

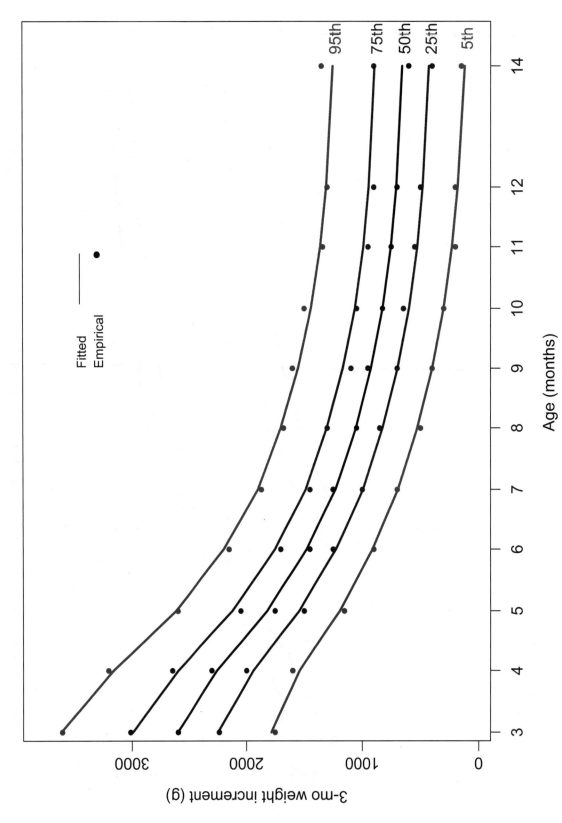

Figure A3.25   5th, 25th, 50th, 75th, 95th smoothed centile curves and empirical values: 3-month weight velocity for girls

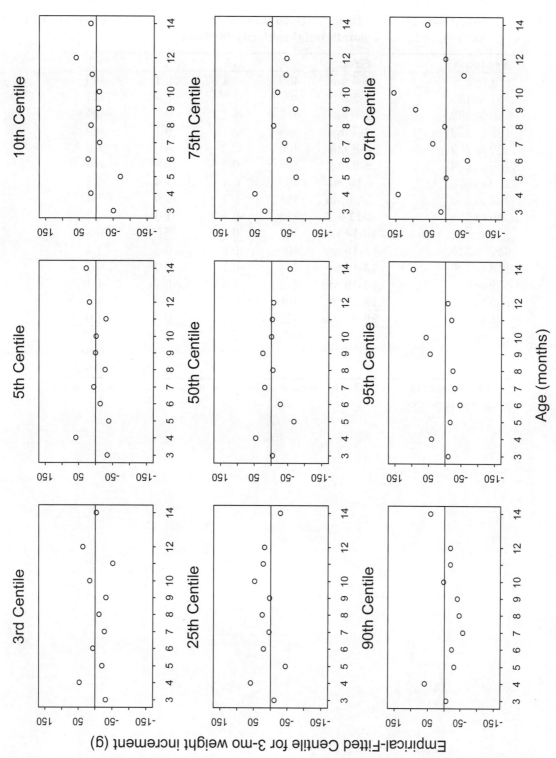

Figure A3.26 Centile residuals from fitting selected model for 3-month weight velocity for girls

A3.4a 4-month intervals for boys

Table A3.5 Q-test for z-scores from selected model [BCPE(x=age$^{0.05}$, df(μ)=11, df(σ)=5, df(ν)=5, τ=2)] for 4-month weight velocity for boys

Age (days)	Group	N	z1	z2	z3
113 to 137	**0-4 mo**	409	-0.4	0.1	0.0
137 to 168	**1-5 mo**	407	1.5	-0.4	0.1
168 to 198	**2-6 mo**	412	-1.1	0.1	-0.4
198 to 229	**3-7 mo**	408	-0.1	0.7	-0.9
229 to 259	**4-8 mo**	400	0.2	0.4	1.0
259 to 289	**5-9 mo**	394	-0.2	-0.8	0.5
289 to 320	**6-10 mo**	395	0.4	-1.4	2.3
320 to 350	**7-11 mo**	406	0.1	-0.9	1.1
350 to 396	**8-12 mo**	396	-0.4	1.3	-1.7
396 to 457	**10-14 mo**	392	0.2	0.9	0.8
457 to 518	**12-16 mo**	400	-0.8	0.7	1.4
518 to 579	**14-18 mo**	404	-0.1	0.7	0.7
579 to 640	**16-20 mo**	413	0.4	-0.7	-1.1
640 to 701	**18-22 mo**	408	0.2	-1.2	1.3
701 to 750	**20-24 mo**	412	-0.1	0.5	1.0
Overall Q stats		6056	5.0	10.0	18.5
degrees of freedom			4.0	12.0	10.0
p-value			0.2898	0.6128	0.0467

Note: Absolute values of z1, z2 or z3 larger than 2 indicate misfit of, respectively, mean, variance or skewness.

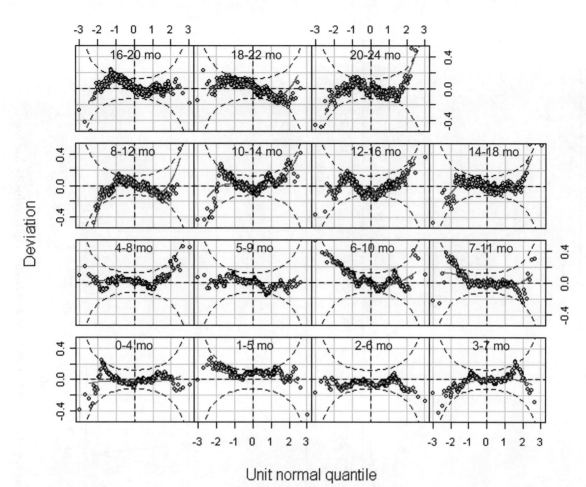

Figure A3.27 Worm plots from selected model [BCPE(x=age$^{0.05}$, df(μ)=11, df(σ)=5, df(ν)=5, τ=2)] for 4-month weight velocity for boys

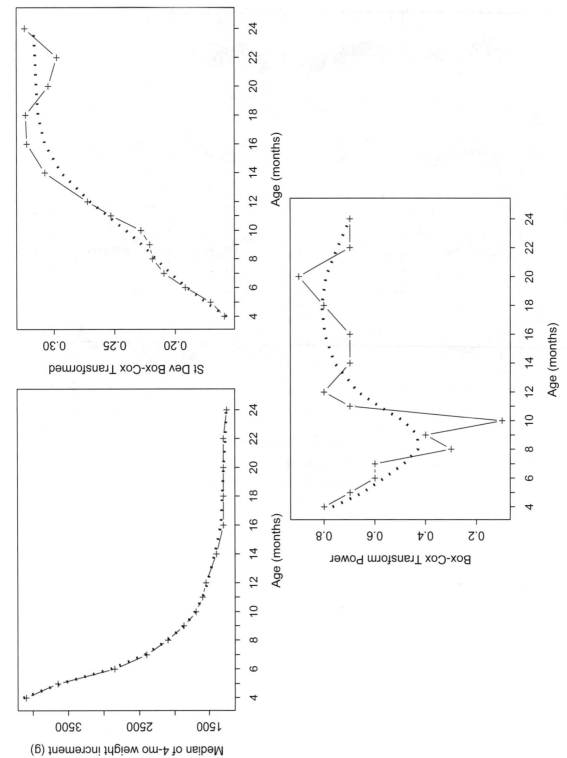

Figure A3.28 Fitting of the μ, σ, and ν curves of selected model for 4-month weight velocity for boys

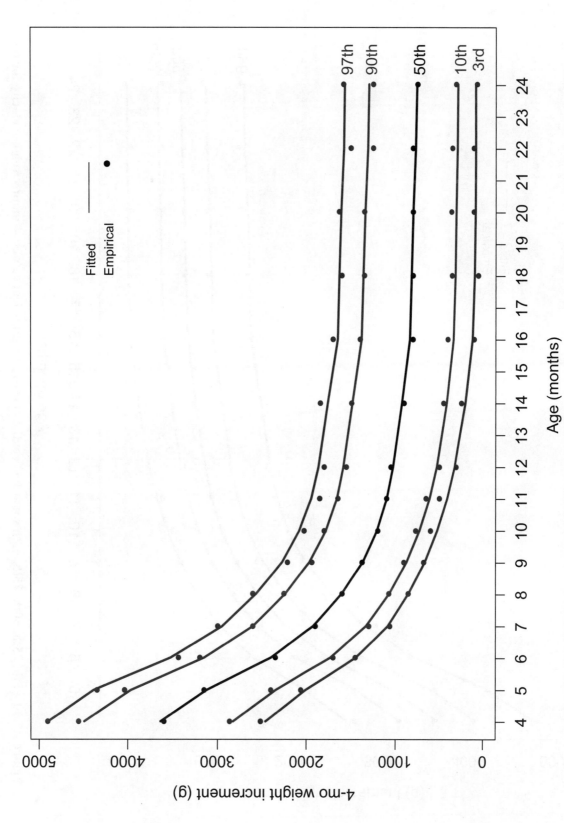

Figure A3.29 3rd, 10th, 50th, 90th, 97th smoothed centile curves and empirical values: 4-month weight velocity for boys

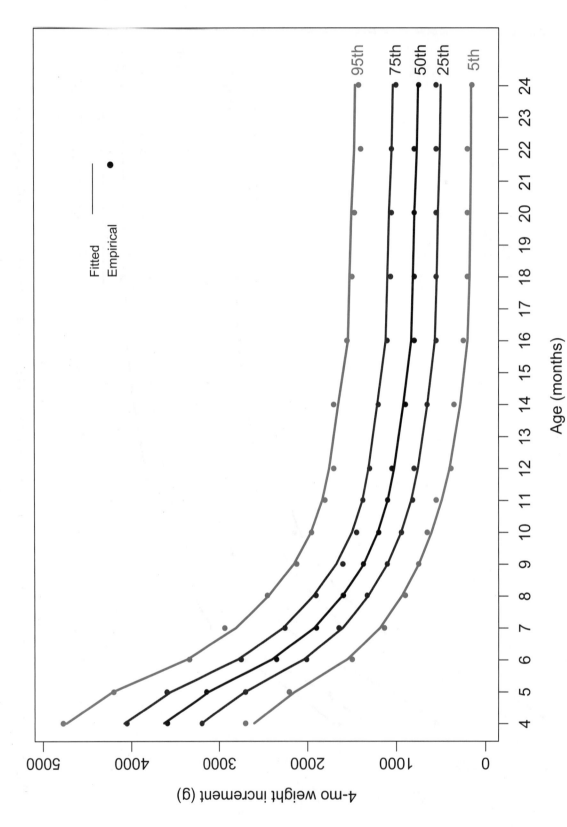

Figure A3.30   5th, 25th, 50th, 75th, 95th smoothed centile curves and empirical values: 4-month weight velocity for boys

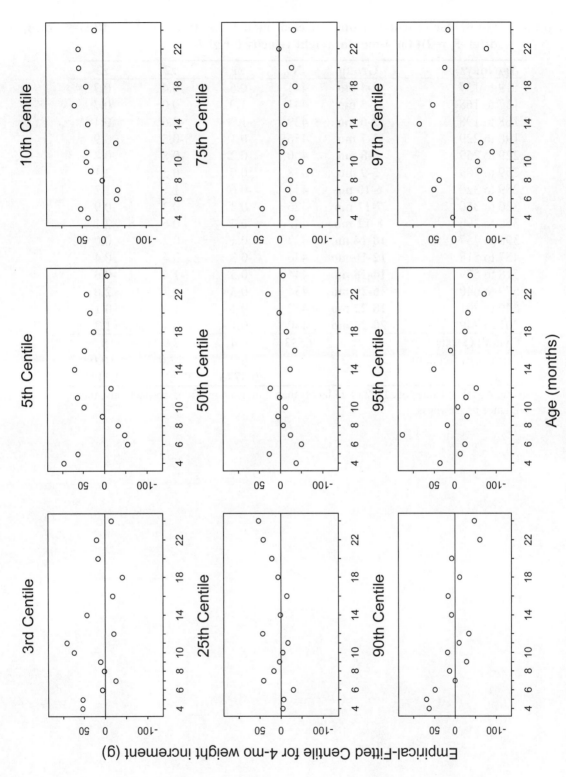

Figure A3.31 Centile residuals from fitting selected model for 4-month weight velocity for boys

A3.4b 4-month intervals for girls

Table A3.6   **Q-test for z-scores from selected model [BCPE(x=age$^{0.05}$, df(μ)=9, df(σ)=5, df(ν)=5, τ=2)] for 4-month weight velocity for girls**

Age (days)	Group	N	z1	z2	z3
119 to 137	**0-4 mo**	441	-0.6	0.4	-0.7
137 to 168	**1-5 mo**	441	1.9	0.0	0.7
168 to 198	**2-6 mo**	439	-1.3	-0.6	0.1
198 to 229	**3-7 mo**	436	0.1	-0.5	0.9
229 to 259	**4-8 mo**	430	0.2	-0.8	0.4
259 to 289	**5-9 mo**	438	0.0	0.3	-2.1
289 to 320	**6-10 mo**	431	-0.6	1.1	1.2
320 to 350	**7-11 mo**	426	0.3	0.3	0.9
350 to 396	**8-12 mo**	432	-0.2	0.6	2.1
396 to 457	**10-14 mo**	433	0.1	-0.2	0.0
457 to 518	**12-16 mo**	436	-0.3	0.4	0.4
518 to 579	**14-18 mo**	444	0.5	-1.4	-0.6
579 to 640	**16-20 mo**	434	0.3	-0.7	2.0
640 to 701	**18-22 mo**	432	-0.1	1.5	-0.1
701 to 749	**20-24 mo**	440	-0.1	-0.4	1.2
Overall Q stats		6533	6.4	7.9	18.7
degrees of freedom			6.0	12.0	10.0
p-value			0.3776	0.7951	0.0441

Note: Absolute values of z1, z2 or z3 larger than 2 indicate misfit of, respectively, mean, variance or skewness.

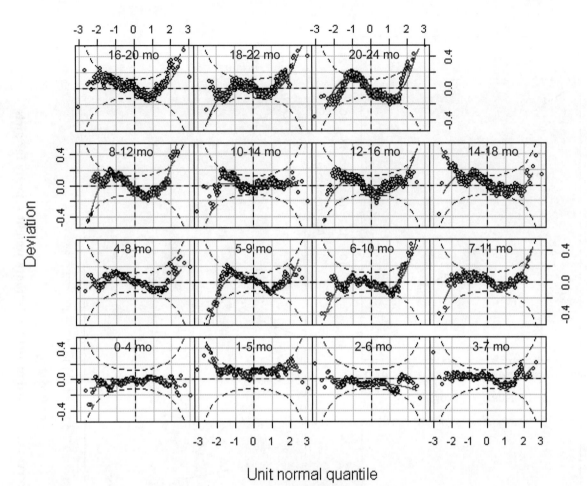

Figure A3.32 Worm plots from selected model [BCPE(x=age$^{0.05}$, df(μ)=9, df(σ)=5, df(ν)=5, τ=2)]
for 4-month weight velocity for girls

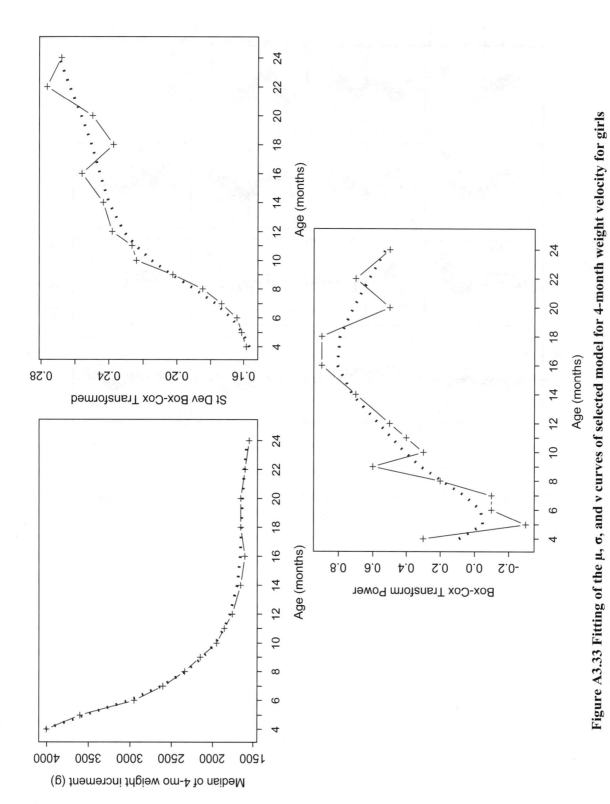

Figure A3.33 Fitting of the μ, σ, and ν curves of selected model for 4-month weight velocity for girls

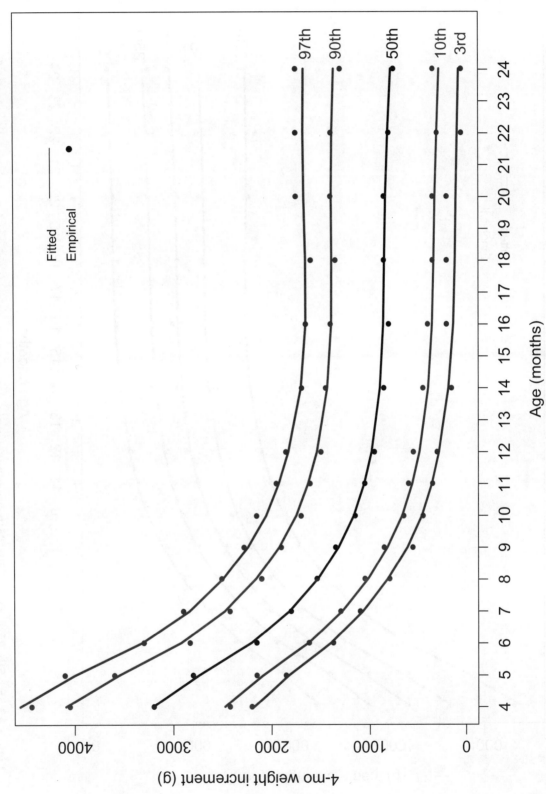

Figure A3.34   3rd, 10th, 50th, 90th, 97th smoothed centile curves and empirical values: 4-month weight velocity for girls

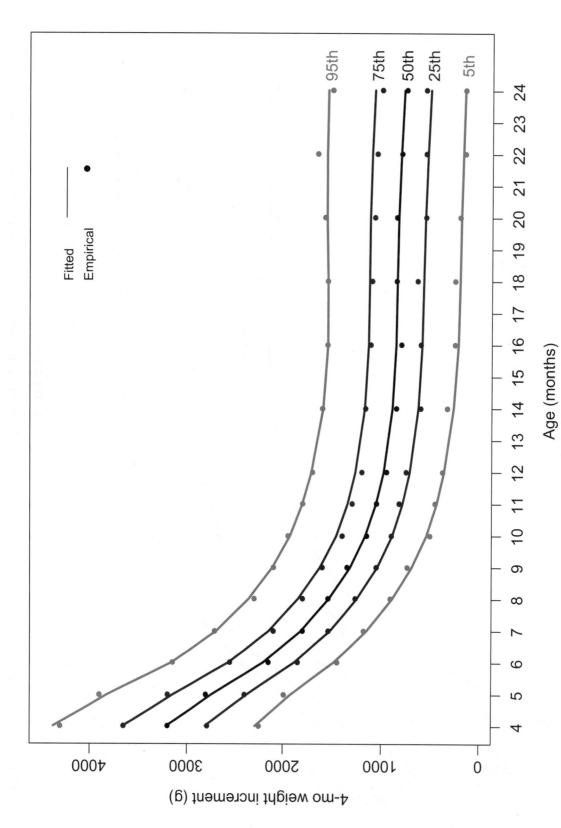

Figure A3.35 5th, 25th, 50th, 75th, 95th smoothed centile curves and empirical values: 4-month weight velocity for girls

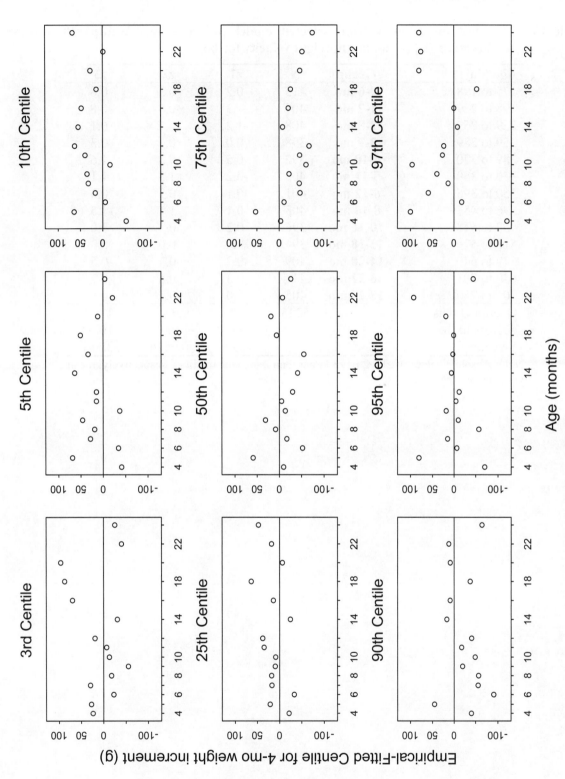

Figure A3.36 Centile residuals from fitting selected model for 4-month weight velocity for girls

A3.5a 6-month intervals for boys

Table A3.7   **Q-test for z-scores from selected model [BCPE(x=age$^{0.05}$, df(μ)=10, df(σ)=5, df(v)=3, τ=2)] for 6-month weight velocity for boys**

Age (days)	Group	N	z1	z2	z3
175 to 198	**0-6 mo**	415	-0.2	-0.3	-0.8
198 to 229	**1-7 mo**	409	1.3	0.5	-0.8
229 to 259	**2-8 mo**	408	-1.2	0.1	0.1
259 to 289	**3-9 mo**	398	0.0	0.1	0.3
289 to 320	**4-10 mo**	392	0.5	-0.3	1.6
320 to 350	**5-11 mo**	405	-0.2	-1.3	1.1
350 to 396	**6-12 mo**	401	0.1	0.3	0.3
396 to 457	**8-14 mo**	403	-0.1	1.1	-1.5
457 to 518	**10-16 mo**	396	-0.2	0.3	3.0
518 to 579	**12-18 mo**	394	0.0	0.0	-0.3
579 to 640	**14-20 mo**	409	-0.2	0.3	-0.5
640 to 701	**16-22 mo**	411	0.3	-0.6	0.7
701 to 750	**18-24 mo**	405	0.0	-0.1	0.8
Overall Q stats		5246	3.5	3.9	17.8
degrees of freedom			3.0	10.0	10.0
p-value			0.3246	0.9516	0.0581

Note: Absolute values of z1, z2 or z3 larger than 2 indicate misfit of, respectively, mean, variance or skewness.

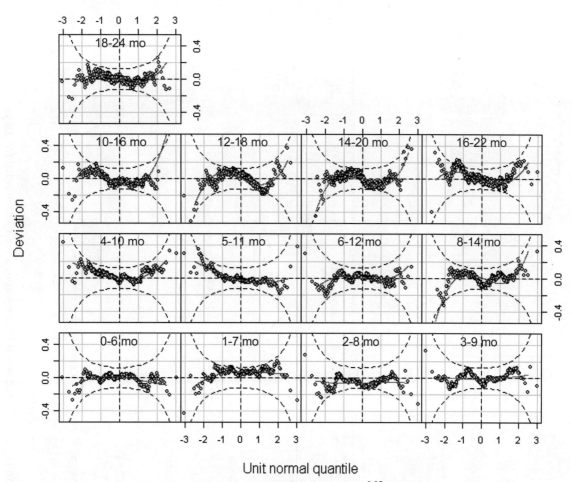

Figure A3.37 Worm plots from selected model [BCPE(x=age$^{0.05}$, df(μ)=10, df(σ)=5, df(ν)=3, τ=2)] for 6-month weight velocity for boys

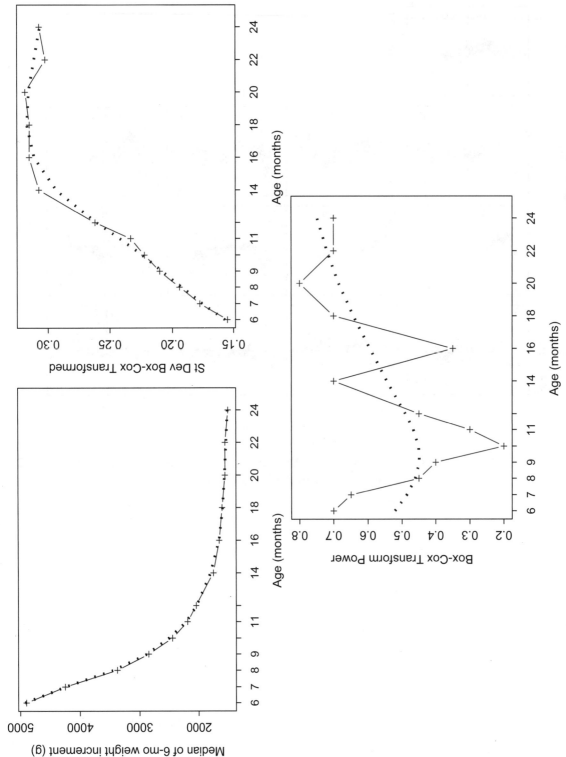

Figure A3.38 Fitting of the μ, σ, and ν curves of selected model for 6-month weight velocity for boys

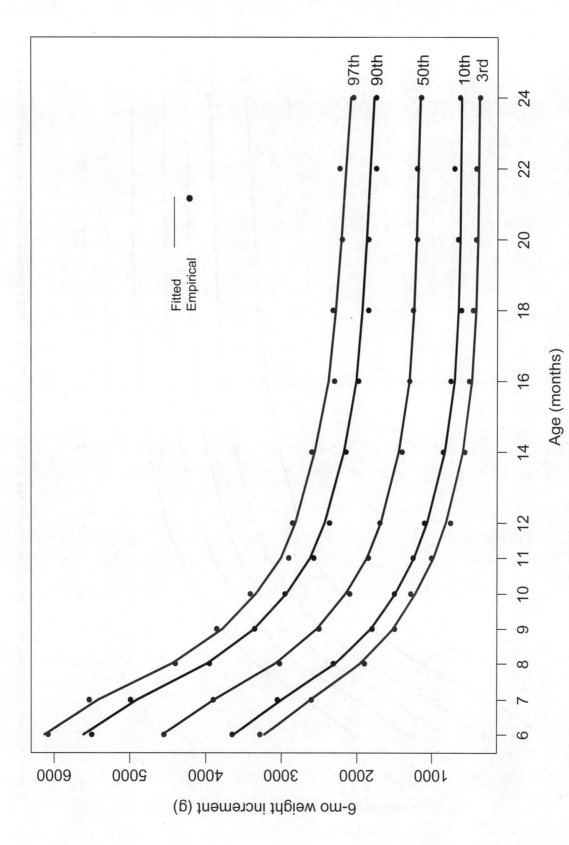

Figure A3.39   **3rd, 10th, 50th, 90th, 97th smoothed centile curves and empirical values: 6-month weight velocity for boys**

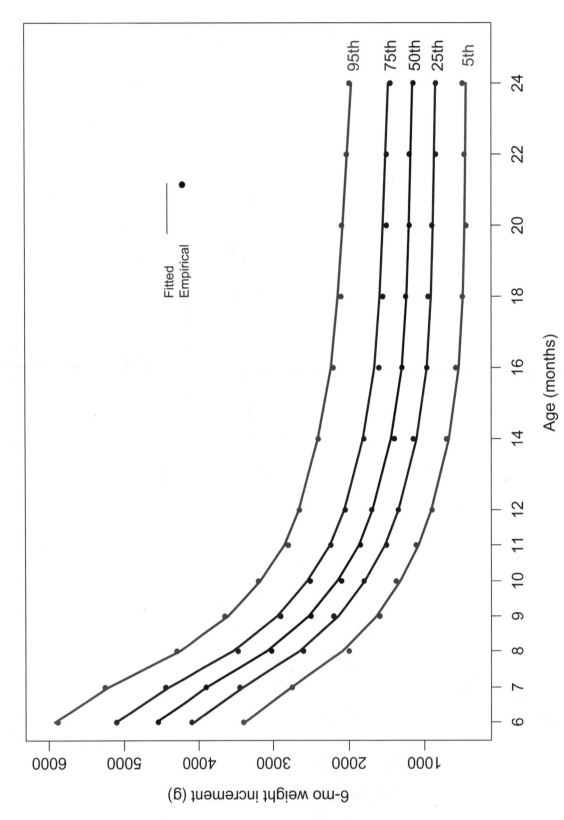

Figure A3.40   5th, 25th, 50th, 75th, 95th smoothed centile curves and empirical values: 6-month weight velocity for boys

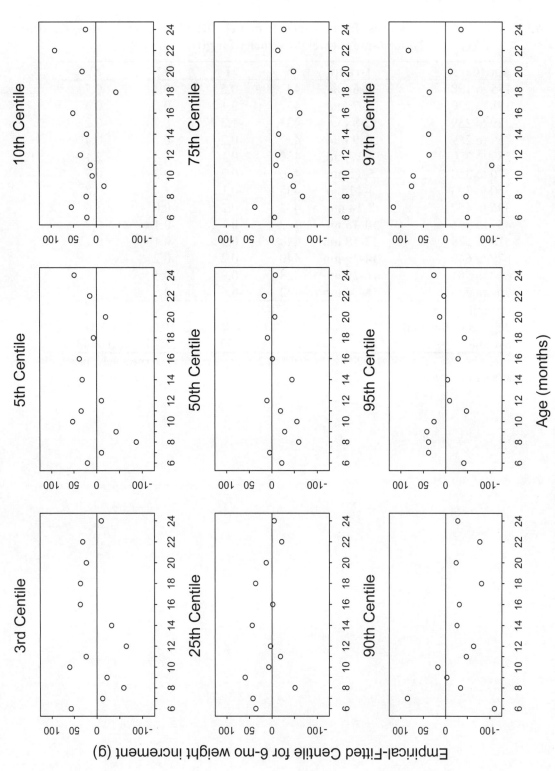

Figure A3.41 Centile residuals from fitting selected model for 6-month weight velocity for boys

A3.5b 6-month intervals for girls

Table A3.8   Q-test for z-scores from selected model [BCPE(x=age$^{0.05}$, df(μ)=7, df(σ)=5, df(v)=4, τ=2)] for 6-month weight velocity for girls

Age (days)	Group	N	z1	z2	z3
175 to 198	**0-6 mo**	442	-0.5	0.4	-0.7
198 to 229	**1-7 mo**	437	2.1	0.0	0.6
229 to 259	**2-8 mo**	433	-1.2	-0.7	-0.2
259 to 289	**3-9 mo**	437	-0.2	-0.5	-0.4
289 to 320	**4-10 mo**	430	-0.1	-0.4	2.1
320 to 350	**5-11 mo**	430	-0.2	0.3	0.7
350 to 396	**6-12 mo**	438	-0.1	1.4	0.8
396 to 457	**8-14 mo**	433	-0.2	0.0	1.0
457 to 518	**10-16 mo**	427	-0.1	-0.1	-0.2
518 to 579	**12-18 mo**	440	0.3	-0.1	0.1
579 to 640	**14-20 mo**	440	-0.2	-0.2	1.5
640 to 701	**16-22 mo**	428	0.9	-0.5	2.7
701 to 750	**18-24 mo**	442	-0.6	0.5	-0.4
Overall Q stats		5657	7.5	3.8	17.3
degrees of freedom			6.0	10.0	9.0
p-value			0.2773	0.9577	0.0448

Note: Absolute values of z1, z2 or z3 larger than 2 indicate misfit of, respectively, mean, variance or skewness.

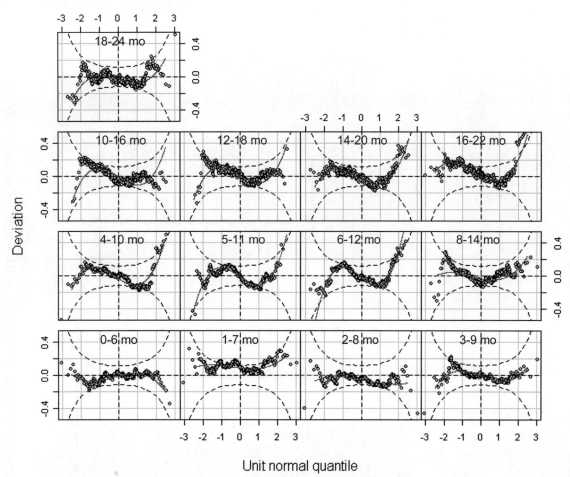

Figure A3.42 Worm plots from selected model [BCPE(x=age$^{0.05}$, df(μ)=7, df(σ)=5, df(ν)=4, τ=2)] for 6-month weight velocity for girls

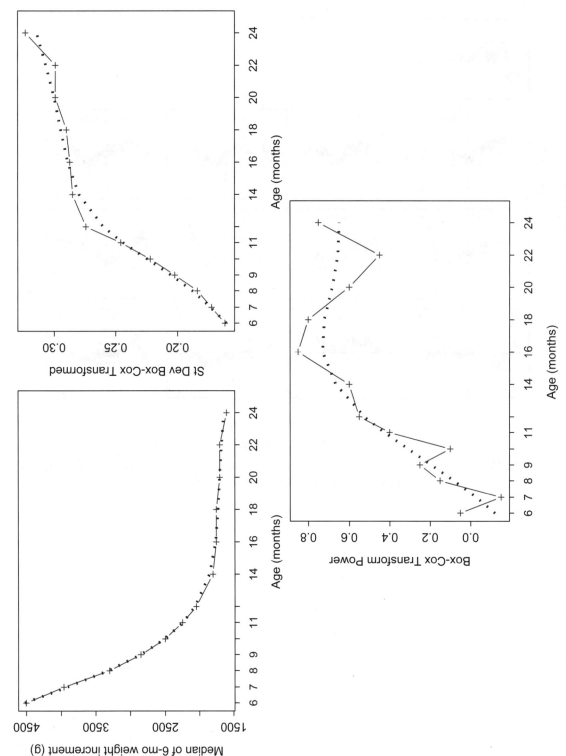

Figure A3.43 Fitting of the μ, σ, and ν curves of selected model for 6-month weight velocity for girls

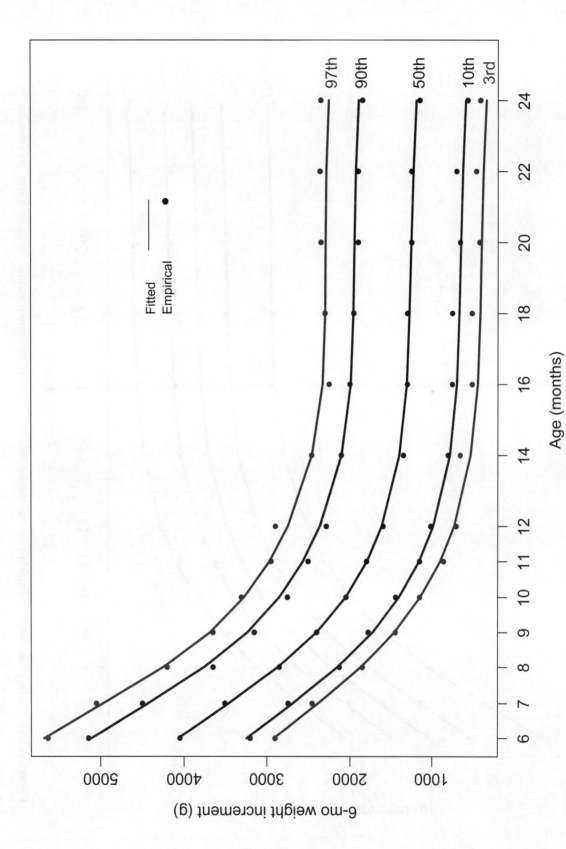

Figure A3.44   3rd, 10th, 50th, 90th, 97th smoothed centile curves and empirical values: 6-month weight velocity for girls

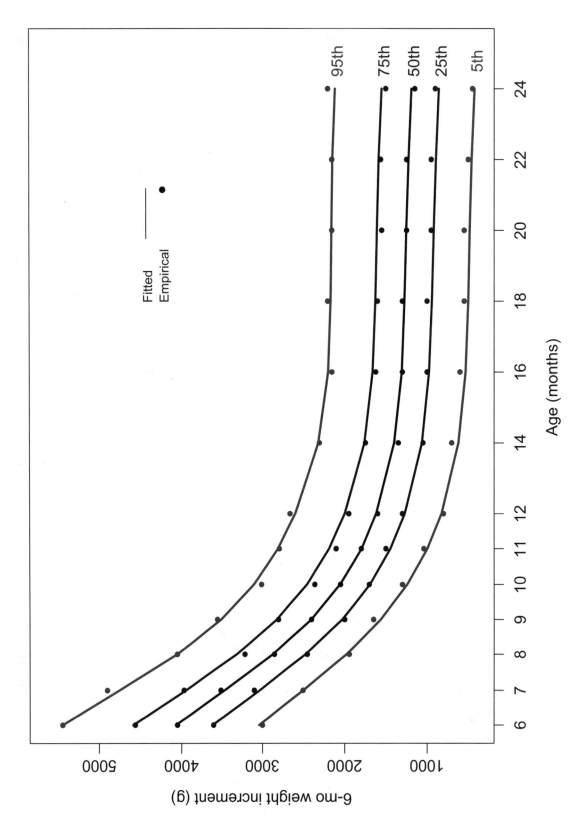

Figure A3.45   5th, 25th, 50th, 75th, 95th smoothed centile curves and empirical values: 6-month weight velocity for girls

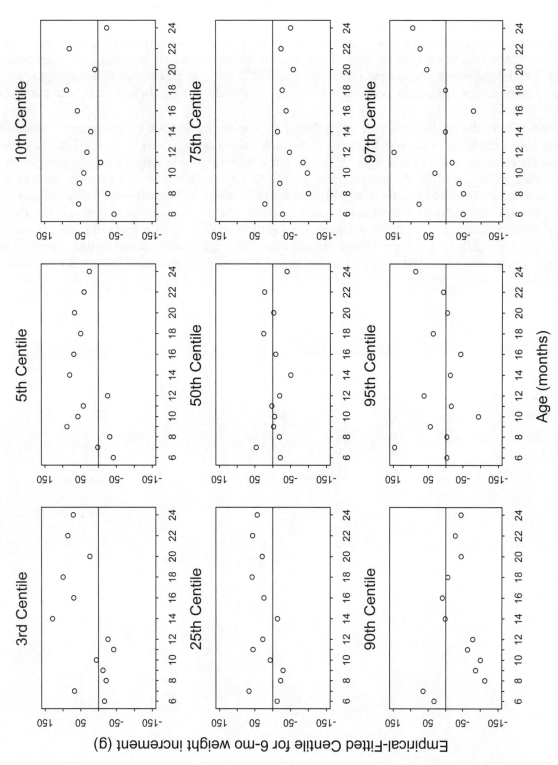

Figure A3.46 Centile residuals from fitting selected model for 6-month weight velocity for girls

3.2   Centile tables of weight velocity by birth weight category from birth to 60 days

This section provides sex-specific centiles for weight increments conditional on birth weight for one- or two-week intervals from birth to 2 months following the MGRS longitudinal component visits schedule. The values are presented both as net increments in grams and as g/day over each index period. The tables, which present the median and the 25th, 10th and 5th centiles that were generated based on empirical estimates, are expected to be particularly useful for lactation management purposes.

The estimation of the centiles was done using the STATA software, which applies a simple method of ranking observations in the sample. The rows of the tables show age intervals in days and the columns provide the grouping of the birth weights in grams. Only the median is provided when the sample size is too small, as happened for the birth-weight group 2 to 2.5 kg. Tables 14 and 16 show the weight gain values by birth-weight group and age interval for boys and girls, respectively. Tables 15 and 17 present the sex-specific daily weight gain values by birth-weight groups and age interval. The daily weight gains, g/d, are not the simple average of the gross gains or losses reported in corresponding weekly and fortnightly tables. Instead, these figures come from calculating individual daily increments for newborns in each of the birth-weight categories and then estimating centiles directly from the raw g/d values.

Table 14   Boys weight increments (g) by birth-weight groups

Age (days)		Birth weight (g)					
		2000-2500	2500-3000	3000-3500	3500-4000	4000+	All
0-7	Median	150	150	150	150	50	150
	25th	-*	0	0	0	-50	0
	10th	-*	-150	-150	-250	-250	-150
	5th	-*	-200	-250	-300	-250	-250
	(n)	(7)	(88)	(142)	(100)	(46)	(383)
7-14	Median	275	250	250	250	275	250
	25th	-*	150	150	100	150	150
	10th	-*	0	50	0	50	0
	5th	-*	-100	-50	-50	-100	-50
	(n)	(6)	(88)	(141)	(100)	(46)	(381)
14-28	Median	600	700	650	700	725	650
	25th	-*	550	550	500	550	550
	10th	-*	450	450	400	400	450
	5th	-*	450	350	350	400	350
	(n)	(7)	(95)	(154)	(113)	(48)	(417)
28-42	Median	600	550	550	550	548	550
	25th	-*	500	450	450	450	450
	10th	-*	350	350	350	300	350
	5th	-*	300	300	300	300	300
	(n)	(7)	(95)	(156)	(113)	(46)	(417)
42-60	Median	450	650	650	650	611	650
	25th	-*	550	500	500	400	500
	10th	-*	450	400	400	300	400
	5th	-*	450	350	350	217	350
	(n)	(7)	(96)	(153)	(113)	(47)	(416)

Note: Results are based on empirical centiles.

*: n is too small to estimate lower centiles.

Table 15   Boys weight velocity (g/d) by birth weight-groups

Age (days)		Birth weight (g)					
		2000-2500	2500-3000	3000-3500	3500-4000	4000+	All
0-7	Median	21	21	21	21	7	21
	25th	-*	0	0	0	-7	0
	10th	-*	-21	-21	-36	-36	-21
	5th	-*	-29	-36	-43	-36	-36
	(n)	(7)	(88)	(142)	(100)	(46)	(383)
7-14	Median	40	36	33	31	36	36
	25th	-*	21	19	14	25	19
	10th	-*	0	6	0	6	0
	5th	-*	-14	-7	-7	-14	-7
	(n)	(6)	(88)	(141)	(100)	(46)	(381)
14-28	Median	43	50	46	50	50	47
	25th	-*	39	39	36	37	38
	10th	-*	34	30	29	33	32
	5th	-*	32	25	23	29	25
	(n)	(7)	(95)	(154)	(113)	(48)	(417)
28-42	Median	40	42	40	41	40	40
	25th	-*	36	31	33	31	32
	10th	-*	27	25	24	21	25
	5th	-*	21	21	21	21	21
	(n)	(7)	(95)	(156)	(113)	(46)	(417)
42-60	Median	24	35	34	34	34	34
	25th	-*	29	28	26	23	28
	10th	-*	25	21	22	15	22
	5th	-*	24	17	19	14	18
	(n)	(7)	(96)	(153)	(113)	(47)	(416)

Note: Results are based on empirical centiles.
    *: n is too small to estimate lower centiles.

Table 16 Girls weight increments (g) by birth-weight groups

Age (days)		2000-2500	2500-3000	3000-3500	3500-4000	4000+	All
				Birth weight (g)			
0-7	Median	0	150	100	100	150	100
	25th	-*	0	0	0	0	0
	10th	-*	-100	-100	-150	-100	-100
	5th	-*	-150	-200	-250	-200	-200
	(n)	(18)	(109)	(147)	(85)	(25)	(384)
7-14	Median	200	200	200	200	200	200
	25th	-*	100	100	100	100	100
	10th	-*	0	0	0	50	0
	5th	-*	-100	-50	-100	0	-50
	(n)	(18)	(108)	(147)	(84)	(25)	(382)
14-28	Median	500	600	550	550	600	550
	25th	-*	450	436	450	450	450
	10th	-*	400	350	300	300	350
	5th	-*	300	300	250	200	300
	(n)	(20)	(124)	(176)	(93)	(28)	(441)
28-42	Median	500	500	465	457	525	500
	25th	-*	382	400	325	375	382
	10th	-*	300	300	295	300	300
	5th	-*	300	250	200	300	250
	(n)	(20)	(127)	(174)	(92)	(28)	(441)
42-60	Median	550	550	500	585	550	550
	25th	-*	400	400	408	334	400
	10th	-*	300	300	350	155	300
	5th	-*	300	289	250	150	288
	(n)	(18)	(127)	(175)	(92)	(28)	(440)

Note: Results are based on empirical centiles.
  *: n is too small to estimate lower centiles.

Table 17   Girls weight velocity (g/d) by birth-weight groups

Age (days)		Birth weight (g)					
		2000-2500	2500-3000	3000-3500	3500-4000	4000+	All
0-7	Median	0	21	14	14	21	14
	25th	-*	0	0	0	0	0
	10th	-*	-14	-14	-21	-14	-14
	5th	-*	-21	-29	-36	-29	-29
	(n)	(18)	(109)	(147)	(85)	(25)	(384)
7-14	Median	29	29	29	29	29	29
	25th	-*	14	14	14	14	14
	10th	-*	0	0	0	7	0
	5th	-*	-12	-7	-14	0	-7
	(n)	(18)	(108)	(147)	(84)	(25)	(382)
14-28	Median	36	43	39	42	44	39
	25th	-*	33	32	32	31	32
	10th	-*	29	25	23	22	25
	5th	-*	21	21	18	17	21
	(n)	(20)	(124)	(176)	(93)	(28)	(441)
28-42	Median	36	36	35	32	38	35
	25th	-*	27	28	25	26	27
	10th	-*	23	21	18	21	21
	5th	-*	21	18	15	21	18
	(n)	(20)	(127)	(174)	(92)	(28)	(441)
42-60	Median	29	31	27	32	29	29
	25th	-*	23	21	23	20	22
	10th	-*	19	18	19	9	18
	5th	-*	17	15	13	9	15
	(n)	(18)	(127)	(175)	(92)	(28)	(440)

Note: Results are based on empirical centiles.
   *: n is too small to estimate lower centiles.

4. CONSTRUCTION OF THE LENGTH VELOCITY STANDARDS

The objective was to create sex-specific velocity curves for 2-, 3-, 4- and 6-month length increments conditional on age. Tables generated from the 2-month increment curves provide estimated centiles for ages 0-2, 1-3, …, 22-24 months; tables generated from the 3-month increment curves provide estimated centiles for ages 0-3, 1-4, …, 21-24 months; tables generated from the 4-month increment curves provide estimated centiles for ages 0-4, 1-5, …, 20-24 months; and tables generated from the 6-month increment curves provide estimated centiles for ages 0-6, 1-7, …, 18-24 months.

Negative length increments are clearly the result of measurement error since children cannot grow shorter. On the strength of biology, therefore, negative increments were recoded as "no growth" by assigning the nominal value of +0.01 to enable their inclusion in the BCPE modelling. The numbers involved were small: for the 2-month increments for boys 11 out of 7016 (0.16%) between -0.5 and -0.05 cm, and for girls 15 out of 7504 (0.20%) between -0.75 and -0.05 cm. To examine if the recoding of these few negative values had an impact on the final centiles, one comparison was made using the girls' 2-month length increments with the negative (adding a delta value to all observations) versus the recoded values. This group was selected since it had a larger number of negative increments. The recoding had no impact on the model specifications and the resulting centiles changed only slightly, by at most 0.1 cm, and for very few cases. At the -3SD, the two models yielded identical estimates for the intervals between birth and 14 months. For the later ages, the analysis including the negative increments resulted in negative centile estimates ranging between -0.1 cm (14-16 months) and -0.5 cm (22-24 months). Treating negative increments as zero growth constrained centile estimates to be zero or above but did not introduce bias. Using the nominal shift to "no growth" thus averted the biological contradiction of expected/predicted negative growth at the extreme low centiles.

4.1 2-month intervals

Boys

There were 7016 2-month length increments for boys, one of which was excluded as an outlier, leaving a final sample of 7015 observations for the modelling exercise. The best value of the age-transformation power was $\lambda=0.05$. The search for the best df(μ) and df(σ) followed, fixing $\lambda=0.05$, $\nu=1$ and $\tau=2$. The model with df(μ)=9 and df(σ)=7 provided the smallest GAIC(3). The next step was to search for the best degrees of freedom to fit the parameter ν for skewness fixing $\tau=2$ and keeping the degrees of freedom for the previously selected μ and σ curves. The smallest GAIC(3) value corresponded to df(ν)=1 and the model BCPE(x=age$^{0.05}$, df(μ)=9, df(σ)=7, df(ν)=1, $\tau=2$) was further evaluated.

The diagnostic results are presented in Appendix A4, section A4.1a. The overall Q-test p-values (Table A4.1) indicate an adequate fit of the parameters μ and σ (p-values > 0.05) yet a significant p-value for the skewness parameter ν. This was caused by residual skewness (absolute z3 values larger than 2) in three out of 17 age groups. The worm plots (Figure A4.1) from this model agree with the Q-test results. By contrast, the fitted curves of the parameters μ, σ and ν seemed adequate when compared to the empirical values (Figure A4.2). The fitted centile curves and empirical centiles, which are shown in figures A4.3 and A4.4, indicate close concordance between the two. Figure A4.5 shows the distribution of empirical minus fitted centile differences with no indication of systematic bias except for a slight under-estimation of the 25th centile by about 0.05 cm.

Table 18 presents the predicted centiles for boys' 2-month length velocities between birth and 24 months.

Girls

There were 7504 2-month length increments for girls. The best value of the age-transformation power was $\lambda=0.05$. The search for the best $df(\mu)$ and $df(\sigma)$ followed, fixing $\lambda=0.05$, $\nu=1$ and $\tau=2$. The model with $df(\mu)=10$ and $df(\sigma)=7$ provided the smallest GAIC(3). The next step was to search for the best degrees of freedom to fit the parameter ν for skewness fixing $\tau=2$ and keeping the degrees of freedom for the previously selected μ and σ curves. The smallest GAIC(3) value corresponded to $df(\nu)=1$ and the model BCPE($x=age^{0.05}$, $df(\mu)=10$, $df(\sigma)=7$, $df(\nu)=1$, $\tau=2$) was further evaluated.

The diagnostic results are presented in Appendix A4, section A4.1b. The Q-test results (Table A4.2) and worm plots (Figure A4.6) indicated an adequate fit of the parameters μ and σ. There were four out of 17 groups with residual skewness, resulting in a significant p-value for the overall test of the ν parameter at level 5%. Furthermore, figure A4.7 displays adequate fitting of the parameters μ and σ, and reasonable smoothing of the fluctuations in the ν parameter when compared with the respective sample estimates: Similar to the boys, comparisons between fitted and empirical centiles and centile residuals depict some patterns of negligible biases usually less than 0.1 cm (Figures A4.8 to A4.10).

Table 19 presents the predicted centiles for girls' 2-month length velocities between birth and 24 months.

4.2   3-month intervals

Boys

There were 4545 3-month length increments for boys, two of which were excluded as outliers, leaving a final sample of 4543 observations for the modelling exercise. The best value of the age-transformation power was $\lambda=0.05$. The search for the best $df(\mu)$ and $df(\sigma)$ followed, fixing $\lambda=0.05$, $\nu=1$ and $\tau=2$. The model with $df(\mu)=7$ and $df(\sigma)=6$ provided the smallest GAIC(3). The next step was to search for the best degrees of freedom to fit the parameter ν for skewness fixing $\tau=2$ and keeping the degrees of freedom for the previously selected μ and σ curves. The smallest GAIC(3) value corresponded to $df(\nu)=1$ and thus the model BCPE($x=age^{0.05}$, $df(\mu)=7$, $df(\sigma)=6$, $df(\nu)=1$, $\tau=2$) was selected to predict the boys' 3-month interval parameter curves up to age 12 months (see step 2 in section 2.5).

Those parameter estimates were joined to their equivalents obtained from the 2- and 4-month interval models (birth to 24 months) and a cubic spline surface was fitted for the μ and σ parameters (M and S). For the L curve, the fitted constant ($df(\nu)=1$ in the model above for the first year) was projected into the second year. The resulting predicted parameter estimates for the 3-month interval (birth to 24 months) from the fitted spline surface (M and S) plus the constant value for L were used to construct the final centiles for the boys' 3-month interval.

The diagnostic test results are presented in Appendix A4, section A4.2a. Figures A4.11 to A4.13 show negligible size bias (of about 0.1 cm over-estimation) comparing the empirical and fitted centiles, and the centile residuals, in the 75th centile and above.

Table 20 presents the predicted centiles for boys' 3-month length velocities between birth and 24 months.

Girls

There were 4866 3-month length increments for girls, one of which was excluded as an outlier, leaving a final sample of 4865 observations for the modelling exercise. The smallest global deviance value corresponded to the age-transformation power $\lambda=0.05$. The search for the best $df(\mu)$ and $df(\sigma)$ followed, fixing $\lambda=0.05$, $\nu=1$ and $\tau=2$. The model with $df(\mu)=8$ and $df(\sigma)=5$ provided the smallest GAIC(3). The next step was to search for the best degrees of freedom to fit the parameter ν for skewness fixing $\tau=2$ and keeping the degrees of freedom for the previously selected μ and σ curves. The smallest GAIC(3) value corresponded to $df(\nu)=1$. The model BCPE($x=age^{0.05}$, $df(\mu)=8$, $df(\sigma)=5$, $df(\nu)=1$, $\tau=2$) was selected to predict the girls' 3-month interval parameter curves up to age 12 months.

Following step 3 of the methodology described in section 2.5, those parameter estimates were joined to their equivalents obtained from the 2- and 4-month interval models (birth to 24 months) for the μ and σ parameters (M and S) and a cubic spline surface was used to fit each of these parameters. Similar to boys, the fitted constant for the ν parameter (L) was projected from the first into the second year. The predicted parameter estimates from the fitted spline surface (M and S) for 3-month interval (birth to 24 months) plus the constant value for L were used to construct the final centiles for the girls' 3-month interval.

The diagnostic test results are presented in Appendix A4, section A4.2b. Comparisons between fitted and empirical centiles (A4.14 and A4.15) and centile residuals (A4.16) show only an average over-estimation smaller than 0.1 cm in the 75th centile.

Table 21 presents the predicted centiles for girls' 3-month weight velocities between birth and 24 months.

4.3 4-month intervals

Boys

There were 6183 4-month length increments for boys. The best value of the age-transformation power was $\lambda=0.05$. The search for the best $df(\mu)$ and $df(\sigma)$ followed, fixing $\lambda=0.05$, $\nu=1$ and $\tau=2$. The model with $df(\mu)=8$ and $df(\sigma)=5$ provided the smallest GAIC(3). The next step was to search for the best degrees of freedom to fit the parameter ν for skewness fixing $\tau=2$ and keeping the degrees of freedom for the previously selected μ and σ curves. The smallest GAIC(3) value corresponded to $df(\nu)=1$, and the model BCPE($x=age^{0.05}$, $df(\mu)=8$, $df(\sigma)=5$, $df(\nu)=1$, $\tau=2$) was further evaluated.

The diagnostic test results are presented in Appendix A4, section A4.3a. The Q-test results (Table A4.3) and worm plots (Figure A4.17) from this model indicated an adequate fit of the data with only 1 out of 15 age groups showing misfit of the median (absolute z1>2) and 2 out of 15 age groups with residual skewness (absolute z3>2). Yet the overall Q-test p-value was non-significant at the 5% level and thus the model was considered adequate. Figure A4.18 shows the fitted μ, σ and ν curves against their corresponding empirical estimates. The ν parameter empirical curve exhibits fluctuations that are reasonably averaged by the fitted value. The next three plots (figures A4.19, A4.20 and A4.21) show no evidence of bias when comparing fitted to empirical centiles or centile residuals, except for a slight under-estimation in the 10th and lower centiles by about 0.1 cm.

Table 22 presents the predicted centiles for boys' 4-month length velocities between birth and 24 months.

Girls

There were 6620 4-month length increments for girls. The best value of the age-transformation power was $\lambda=0.05$. The search for the best $df(\mu)$ and $df(\sigma)$ followed, fixing $\lambda=0.05$, $\nu=1$ and $\tau=2$. The model with $df(\mu)=8$ and $df(\sigma)=5$ provided the smallest GAIC(3). The next step was to search for the best degrees of freedom to fit the parameter ν for skewness fixing $\tau=2$ and keeping the degrees of freedom for the previously selected μ and σ curves. The smallest GAIC(3) value corresponded to $df(\nu)=1$ and the model BCPE($x=age^{0.05}$, $df(\mu)=8$, $df(\sigma)=5$, $df(\nu)=1$, $\tau=2$) was further evaluated.

The diagnostic results are presented in Appendix A4, section A4.3b. The Q-test results (Table A4.4) and worm plots (Figure A4.22) from this model indicated clearly that it was adequate for constructing the 4-month velocity curves for girls. Figure A4.23 shows adequate fitting of the parameters μ and σ with the respective sample estimates and a fair constant fitting of the fluctuations in the empirical curve for ν by the selected model. Comparisons between fitted and empirical centiles and centile residuals depict a reasonable fit of the data with a slight over-estimation in the 75th centile by about 0.05 cm (Figures A4.24 to A4.26).

Table 23 presents the predicted centiles for girls' 4-month length velocities between birth and 24 months.

4.4   6-month intervals

Boys

There were a total of 5358 6-month length increments for boys, one of which was excluded as an outlier, leaving a final sample of 5357 increments for the modelling exercise. The best value of the age-transformation power was $\lambda=0.05$. The search for the best $df(\mu)$ and $df(\sigma)$ followed, fixing $\lambda=0.05$, $\nu=1$ and $\tau=2$. The model with $df(\mu)=7$ and $df(\sigma)=5$ corresponded to the smallest GAIC(3). The next step was to search for the best degrees of freedom to fit the parameter ν for skewness fixing $\tau=2$ and keeping the degrees of freedom for the previously selected μ and σ curves. Although the smallest GAIC(3) value corresponded to $df(\nu)=3$, the model with $df(\nu)=1$ was also considered to be more consistent with the other intervals. Since there were no detectable differences in the final centiles estimated by either model, the simpler model (i.e. BCPE($x=age^{0.05}$, $df(\mu)=7$, $df(\sigma)=5$, $df(\nu)=1$, $\tau=2$) was further evaluated.

The diagnostic test results are presented in the Appendix A4, section A4.4a. The Q-test results (Table A4.5) and worm plots (Figure A4.27) from this model indicated an adequate fit of the data with only 1 out of 13 age groups showing misfit of the skewness (absolute z3>2). Yet the overall Q-test p-value was non-significant at the 5% level and thus the model was considered adequate. Figure A4.28 shows the fitted μ, σ and ν curves against their corresponding empirical estimates. The ν parameter empirical curve fluctuated and was well averaged by the fitted constant value. The next three plots (figures A4.29, A4.30 and A4.31) show no evidence of bias when comparing fitted to empirical centiles or centile residuals, except for a slight over-estimation by about 0.1 cm in the 90th and 95th centiles.

Table 24 presents the predicted centiles for boys' 6-month length velocities between birth and 24 months.

Girls

There were 5739 6-month length increments for girls. The best value of the age-transformation power was $\lambda=0.05$. The search for the best df(μ) and df(σ) followed, fixing $\lambda=0.05$, $v=1$ and $\tau=2$. The model with df(μ)=7 and df(σ)=4 provided the smallest GAIC(3). The next step was to search for the best degrees of freedom to fit the parameter v for skewness fixing $\tau=2$ and keeping the degrees of freedom for the previously selected μ and σ curves. The smallest GAIC(3) value corresponded to df(v)=1 and the model BCPE(x=age$^{0.05}$, df(μ)=7, df(σ)=4, df(v)=1, $\tau=2$) was further evaluated.

The diagnostic results are presented in Appendix A4, section A4.4b. The Q-test results (Table A4.6) and worm plots (Figure A4.32) from this model indicated clearly that it was adequate for constructing the 6-month velocity curves for girls. Figure A4.33 shows adequate fitting of the parameters μ and σ curves with the respective sample estimates. The fluctuations in the empirical curve for v are fitted reasonably well by the constant in the selected model. Comparisons between fitted and empirical centiles and centile residuals depict fair concordance between the empirical and fitted data (Figures A4.34 to A4.36).

Table 25 presents the predicted centiles for girls' 6-month length velocities between birth and 24 months.

Table 18 Boys 2-month length increments (cm)

Interval	L	M	S	1st	3rd	5th	15th	25th	50th	75th	85th	95th	97th	99th
0-2 mo	0.9497	8.4820	0.13400	5.9	6.4	6.6	7.3	7.7	8.5	9.3	9.7	10.4	10.6	11.1
1-3 mo	0.9497	6.9984	0.14062	4.7	5.2	5.4	6.0	6.3	7.0	7.7	8.0	8.6	8.9	9.3
2-4 mo	0.9497	5.5716	0.17179	3.4	3.8	4.0	4.6	4.9	5.6	6.2	6.6	7.2	7.4	7.8
3-5 mo	0.9497	4.4941	0.20929	2.3	2.7	3.0	3.5	3.9	4.5	5.1	5.5	6.1	6.3	6.7
4-6 mo	0.9497	3.7228	0.24323	1.7	2.0	2.3	2.8	3.1	3.7	4.3	4.7	5.2	5.4	5.9
5-7 mo	0.9497	3.2403	0.26837	1.3	1.6	1.8	2.3	2.7	3.2	3.8	4.1	4.7	4.9	5.3
6-8 mo	0.9497	2.9661	0.28481	1.0	1.4	1.6	2.1	2.4	3.0	3.5	3.8	4.4	4.6	5.0
7-9 mo	0.9497	2.8089	0.29636	0.9	1.3	1.5	2.0	2.3	2.8	3.4	3.7	4.2	4.4	4.8
8-10 mo	0.9497	2.6901	0.30505	0.8	1.2	1.4	1.8	2.1	2.7	3.2	3.5	4.1	4.3	4.6
9-11 mo	0.9497	2.5785	0.31391	0.7	1.1	1.3	1.7	2.0	2.6	3.1	3.4	3.9	4.1	4.5
10-12 mo	0.9497	2.4724	0.32400	0.7	1.0	1.2	1.7	1.9	2.5	3.0	3.3	3.8	4.0	4.4
11-13 mo	0.9497	2.3818	0.33613	0.6	0.9	1.1	1.6	1.8	2.4	2.9	3.2	3.7	3.9	4.3
12-14 mo	0.9497	2.2978	0.34908	0.5	0.8	1.0	1.5	1.8	2.3	2.8	3.1	3.6	3.8	4.2
13-15 mo	0.9497	2.2138	0.36174	0.4	0.7	0.9	1.4	1.7	2.2	2.8	3.1	3.5	3.7	4.1
14-16 mo	0.9497	2.1357	0.37410	0.3	0.7	0.8	1.3	1.6	2.1	2.7	3.0	3.5	3.7	4.0
15-17 mo	0.9497	2.0675	0.38645	0.3	0.6	0.8	1.2	1.5	2.1	2.6	2.9	3.4	3.6	4.0
16-18 mo	0.9497	2.0061	0.39924	0.2	0.5	0.7	1.2	1.5	2.0	2.5	2.8	3.3	3.5	3.9
17-19 mo	0.9497	1.9495	0.41274	0.2	0.5	0.7	1.1	1.4	1.9	2.5	2.8	3.3	3.5	3.9
18-20 mo	0.9497	1.8972	0.42656	0.1	0.4	0.6	1.1	1.4	1.9	2.4	2.7	3.2	3.4	3.8
19-21 mo	0.9497	1.8490	0.44029	0.0	0.4	0.5	1.0	1.3	1.8	2.4	2.7	3.2	3.4	3.8
20-22 mo	0.9497	1.8030	0.45398	0.0	0.3	0.5	1.0	1.3	1.8	2.4	2.7	3.2	3.4	3.7
21-23 mo	0.9497	1.7575	0.46768	0.0	0.3	0.4	0.9	1.2	1.8	2.3	2.6	3.1	3.3	3.7
22-24 mo	0.9497	1.7133	0.48129	0.0	0.2	0.4	0.9	1.2	1.7	2.3	2.6	3.1	3.3	3.7

Table 18   Boys 2-month length increments (cm) - *continued*

Interval	L	M	S	-3SD	-2SD	-1SD	Median	+1SD	+2SD	+3SD
0-2 mo	0.9497	8.4820	0.13400	5.1	6.2	7.3	8.5	9.6	10.8	11.9
1-3 mo	0.9497	6.9984	0.14062	4.1	5.0	6.0	7.0	8.0	9.0	10.0
2-4 mo	0.9497	5.5716	0.17179	2.7	3.7	4.6	5.6	6.5	7.5	8.5
3-5 mo	0.9497	4.4941	0.20929	1.7	2.6	3.6	4.5	5.4	6.4	7.4
4-6 mo	0.9497	3.7228	0.24323	1.1	1.9	2.8	3.7	4.6	5.6	6.5
5-7 mo	0.9497	3.2403	0.26837	0.7	1.5	2.4	3.2	4.1	5.0	5.9
6-8 mo	0.9497	2.9661	0.28481	0.5	1.3	2.1	3.0	3.8	4.7	5.5
7-9 mo	0.9497	2.8089	0.29636	0.4	1.2	2.0	2.8	3.6	4.5	5.4
8-10 mo	0.9497	2.6901	0.30505	0.3	1.1	1.9	2.7	3.5	4.4	5.2
9-11 mo	0.9497	2.5785	0.31391	0.2	1.0	1.8	2.6	3.4	4.2	5.1
10-12 mo	0.9497	2.4724	0.32400	0.2	0.9	1.7	2.5	3.3	4.1	4.9
11-13 mo	0.9497	2.3818	0.33613	0.1	0.8	1.6	2.4	3.2	4.0	4.8
12-14 mo	0.9497	2.2978	0.34908	0.0	0.7	1.5	2.3	3.1	3.9	4.8
13-15 mo	0.9497	2.2138	0.36174	0.0	0.7	1.4	2.2	3.0	3.8	4.7
14-16 mo	0.9497	2.1357	0.37410	0.0	0.6	1.3	2.1	2.9	3.8	4.6
15-17 mo	0.9497	2.0675	0.38645	0.0	0.5	1.3	2.1	2.9	3.7	4.5
16-18 mo	0.9497	2.0061	0.39924	0.0	0.4	1.2	2.0	2.8	3.6	4.5
17-19 mo	0.9497	1.9495	0.41274	0.0	0.4	1.2	1.9	2.8	3.6	4.4
18-20 mo	0.9497	1.8972	0.42656	0.0	0.3	1.1	1.9	2.7	3.5	4.4
19-21 mo	0.9497	1.8490	0.44029	0.0	0.3	1.0	1.8	2.7	3.5	4.4
20-22 mo	0.9497	1.8030	0.45398	0.0	0.2	1.0	1.8	2.6	3.5	4.3
21-23 mo	0.9497	1.7575	0.46768	0.0	0.2	0.9	1.8	2.6	3.4	4.3
22-24 mo	0.9497	1.7133	0.48129	0.0	0.1	0.9	1.7	2.5	3.4	4.3

Table 19 Girls 2-month length increments (cm)

Interval	L	M	S	1st	3rd	5th	15th	25th	50th	75th	85th	95th	97th	99th
0-2 mo	0.9918	7.9023	0.14123	5.3	5.8	6.1	6.7	7.1	7.9	8.7	9.1	9.7	10.0	10.5
1-3 mo	0.9918	6.3775	0.15004	4.2	4.6	4.8	5.4	5.7	6.4	7.0	7.4	8.0	8.2	8.6
2-4 mo	0.9918	5.1574	0.17732	3.0	3.4	3.7	4.2	4.5	5.2	5.8	6.1	6.7	6.9	7.3
3-5 mo	0.9918	4.2877	0.21092	2.2	2.6	2.8	3.4	3.7	4.3	4.9	5.2	5.8	6.0	6.4
4-6 mo	0.9918	3.5965	0.23941	1.6	2.0	2.2	2.7	3.0	3.6	4.2	4.5	5.0	5.2	5.6
5-7 mo	0.9918	3.1827	0.25995	1.3	1.6	1.8	2.3	2.6	3.2	3.7	4.0	4.5	4.7	5.1
6-8 mo	0.9918	3.0000	0.27597	1.1	1.4	1.6	2.1	2.4	3.0	3.6	3.9	4.4	4.6	4.9
7-9 mo	0.9918	2.8764	0.28638	1.0	1.3	1.5	2.0	2.3	2.9	3.4	3.7	4.2	4.4	4.8
8-10 mo	0.9918	2.7444	0.29192	0.9	1.2	1.4	1.9	2.2	2.7	3.3	3.6	4.1	4.3	4.6
9-11 mo	0.9918	2.6284	0.29751	0.8	1.2	1.3	1.8	2.1	2.6	3.2	3.4	3.9	4.1	4.5
10-12 mo	0.9918	2.5303	0.30553	0.7	1.1	1.3	1.7	2.0	2.5	3.1	3.3	3.8	4.0	4.3
11-13 mo	0.9918	2.4425	0.31612	0.7	1.0	1.2	1.6	1.9	2.4	3.0	3.2	3.7	3.9	4.2
12-14 mo	0.9918	2.3621	0.32828	0.6	0.9	1.1	1.6	1.8	2.4	2.9	3.2	3.6	3.8	4.2
13-15 mo	0.9918	2.2879	0.34112	0.5	0.8	1.0	1.5	1.8	2.3	2.8	3.1	3.6	3.8	4.1
14-16 mo	0.9918	2.2236	0.35425	0.4	0.7	0.9	1.4	1.7	2.2	2.8	3.0	3.5	3.7	4.1
15-17 mo	0.9918	2.1684	0.36737	0.3	0.7	0.9	1.3	1.6	2.2	2.7	3.0	3.5	3.7	4.0
16-18 mo	0.9918	2.1113	0.38003	0.3	0.6	0.8	1.3	1.6	2.1	2.7	2.9	3.4	3.6	4.0
17-19 mo	0.9918	2.0470	0.39199	0.2	0.5	0.7	1.2	1.5	2.0	2.6	2.9	3.4	3.6	3.9
18-20 mo	0.9918	1.9822	0.40358	0.1	0.5	0.7	1.2	1.4	2.0	2.5	2.8	3.3	3.5	3.8
19-21 mo	0.9918	1.9225	0.41519	0.1	0.4	0.6	1.1	1.4	1.9	2.5	2.8	3.2	3.4	3.8
20-22 mo	0.9918	1.8682	0.42686	0.0	0.4	0.6	1.0	1.3	1.9	2.4	2.7	3.2	3.4	3.7
21-23 mo	0.9918	1.8192	0.43859	0.0	0.3	0.5	1.0	1.3	1.8	2.4	2.6	3.1	3.3	3.7
22-24 mo	0.9918	1.7750	0.45033	0.0	0.3	0.5	0.9	1.2	1.8	2.3	2.6	3.1	3.3	3.6

Table 19 Girls 2-month length increments (cm) - *continued*

Interval	L	M	S	-3SD	-2SD	-1SD	Median	+1SD	+2SD	+3SD
0-2 mo	0.9918	7.9023	0.14123	4.6	5.7	6.8	7.9	9.0	10.1	11.3
1-3 mo	0.9918	6.3775	0.15004	3.5	4.5	5.4	6.4	7.3	8.3	9.3
2-4 mo	0.9918	5.1574	0.17732	2.4	3.3	4.2	5.2	6.1	7.0	7.9
3-5 mo	0.9918	4.2877	0.21092	1.6	2.5	3.4	4.3	5.2	6.1	7.0
4-6 mo	0.9918	3.5965	0.23941	1.0	1.9	2.7	3.6	4.5	5.3	6.2
5-7 mo	0.9918	3.1827	0.25995	0.7	1.5	2.4	3.2	4.0	4.8	5.7
6-8 mo	0.9918	3.0000	0.27597	0.5	1.3	2.2	3.0	3.8	4.7	5.5
7-9 mo	0.9918	2.8764	0.28638	0.4	1.2	2.1	2.9	3.7	4.5	5.4
8-10 mo	0.9918	2.7444	0.29192	0.4	1.1	1.9	2.7	3.5	4.3	5.2
9-11 mo	0.9918	2.6284	0.29751	0.3	1.1	1.8	2.6	3.4	4.2	5.0
10-12 mo	0.9918	2.5303	0.30553	0.2	1.0	1.8	2.5	3.3	4.1	4.9
11-13 mo	0.9918	2.4425	0.31612	0.1	0.9	1.7	2.4	3.2	4.0	4.8
12-14 mo	0.9918	2.3621	0.32828	0.1	0.8	1.6	2.4	3.1	3.9	4.7
13-15 mo	0.9918	2.2879	0.34112	0.1	0.7	1.5	2.3	3.1	3.9	4.6
14-16 mo	0.9918	2.2236	0.35425	0.1	0.7	1.4	2.2	3.0	3.8	4.6
15-17 mo	0.9918	2.1684	0.36737	0.1	0.6	1.4	2.2	3.0	3.8	4.6
16-18 mo	0.9918	2.1113	0.38003	0.1	0.5	1.3	2.1	2.9	3.7	4.5
17-19 mo	0.9918	2.0470	0.39199	0.1	0.4	1.2	2.0	2.9	3.7	4.5
18-20 mo	0.9918	1.9822	0.40358	0.1	0.4	1.2	2.0	2.8	3.6	4.4
19-21 mo	0.9918	1.9225	0.41519	0.1	0.3	1.1	1.9	2.7	3.5	4.3
20-22 mo	0.9918	1.8682	0.42686	0.0	0.3	1.1	1.9	2.7	3.5	4.3
21-23 mo	0.9918	1.8192	0.43859	0.0	0.2	1.0	1.8	2.6	3.4	4.2
22-24 mo	0.9918	1.7750	0.45033	0.0	0.2	1.0	1.8	2.6	3.4	4.2

Table 20 Boys 3-month length increments (cm)

Interval	L	M	S	1st	3rd	5th	15th	25th	50th	75th	85th	95th	97th	99th
0-3 mo	0.8792	11.4458	0.11285	8.5	9.0	9.3	10.1	10.6	11.4	12.3	12.8	13.6	13.9	14.5
1-4 mo	0.8792	9.4950	0.12700	6.7	7.3	7.5	8.3	8.7	9.5	10.3	10.8	11.5	11.8	12.3
2-5 mo	0.8792	7.6058	0.15474	4.9	5.4	5.7	6.4	6.8	7.6	8.4	8.8	9.6	9.9	10.4
3-6 mo	0.8792	6.2317	0.18096	3.7	4.2	4.4	5.1	5.5	6.2	7.0	7.4	8.1	8.4	8.9
4-7 mo	0.8792	5.3243	0.20103	2.9	3.4	3.6	4.2	4.6	5.3	6.1	6.4	7.1	7.4	7.9
5-8 mo	0.8792	4.7433	0.21513	2.5	2.9	3.1	3.7	4.1	4.7	5.4	5.8	6.5	6.7	7.2
6-9 mo	0.8792	4.3594	0.22535	2.2	2.6	2.8	3.4	3.7	4.4	5.0	5.4	6.0	6.3	6.7
7-10 mo	0.8792	4.1002	0.23308	2.0	2.4	2.6	3.1	3.5	4.1	4.8	5.1	5.7	5.9	6.4
8-11 mo	0.8792	3.9200	0.23935	1.8	2.2	2.4	3.0	3.3	3.9	4.6	4.9	5.5	5.7	6.2
9-12 mo	0.8792	3.7818	0.24526	1.7	2.1	2.3	2.8	3.2	3.8	4.4	4.8	5.3	5.6	6.0
10-13 mo	0.8792	3.6611	0.25157	1.6	2.0	2.2	2.7	3.0	3.7	4.3	4.6	5.2	5.4	5.9
11-14 mo	0.8792	3.5430	0.25876	1.5	1.9	2.1	2.6	2.9	3.5	4.2	4.5	5.1	5.3	5.7
12-15 mo	0.8792	3.4189	0.26713	1.4	1.8	2.0	2.5	2.8	3.4	4.0	4.4	5.0	5.2	5.6
13-16 mo	0.8792	3.2920	0.27641	1.3	1.6	1.8	2.4	2.7	3.3	3.9	4.3	4.8	5.1	5.5
14-17 mo	0.8792	3.1717	0.28590	1.2	1.5	1.7	2.3	2.6	3.2	3.8	4.1	4.7	4.9	5.4
15-18 mo	0.8792	3.0649	0.29508	1.1	1.4	1.6	2.1	2.5	3.1	3.7	4.0	4.6	4.8	5.2
16-19 mo	0.8792	2.9758	0.30351	1.0	1.3	1.5	2.1	2.4	3.0	3.6	3.9	4.5	4.7	5.2
17-20 mo	0.8792	2.9068	0.31089	0.9	1.3	1.5	2.0	2.3	2.9	3.5	3.9	4.4	4.7	5.1
18-21 mo	0.8792	2.8507	0.31767	0.9	1.2	1.4	1.9	2.2	2.9	3.5	3.8	4.4	4.6	5.0
19-22 mo	0.8792	2.7940	0.32487	0.8	1.2	1.4	1.9	2.2	2.8	3.4	3.8	4.3	4.6	5.0
20-23 mo	0.8792	2.7265	0.33332	0.7	1.1	1.3	1.8	2.1	2.7	3.3	3.7	4.3	4.5	4.9
21-24 mo	0.8792	2.6405	0.34377	0.7	1.0	1.2	1.7	2.0	2.6	3.3	3.6	4.2	4.4	4.8

Table 20 Boys 3-month length increments (cm) - *continued*

Interval	L	M	S	-3SD	-2SD	-1SD	Median	+1SD	+2SD	+3SD
0-3 mo	0.8792	11.4458	0.11285	7.7	8.9	10.2	11.4	12.7	14.1	15.4
1-4 mo	0.8792	9.4950	0.12700	6.0	7.1	8.3	9.5	10.7	11.9	13.2
2-5 mo	0.8792	7.6058	0.15474	4.2	5.3	6.4	7.6	8.8	10.0	11.2
3-6 mo	0.8792	6.2317	0.18096	3.0	4.0	5.1	6.2	7.4	8.5	9.7
4-7 mo	0.8792	5.3243	0.20103	2.3	3.2	4.3	5.3	6.4	7.5	8.6
5-8 mo	0.8792	4.7433	0.21513	1.8	2.8	3.7	4.7	5.8	6.8	7.9
6-9 mo	0.8792	4.3594	0.22535	1.6	2.5	3.4	4.4	5.4	6.4	7.4
7-10 mo	0.8792	4.1002	0.23308	1.4	2.3	3.2	4.1	5.1	6.1	7.1
8-11 mo	0.8792	3.9200	0.23935	1.3	2.1	3.0	3.9	4.9	5.8	6.8
9-12 mo	0.8792	3.7818	0.24526	1.2	2.0	2.9	3.8	4.7	5.7	6.7
10-13 mo	0.8792	3.6611	0.25157	1.1	1.9	2.8	3.7	4.6	5.6	6.5
11-14 mo	0.8792	3.5430	0.25876	1.0	1.8	2.6	3.5	4.5	5.4	6.4
12-15 mo	0.8792	3.4189	0.26713	0.9	1.7	2.5	3.4	4.3	5.3	6.3
13-16 mo	0.8792	3.2920	0.27641	0.7	1.5	2.4	3.3	4.2	5.2	6.1
14-17 mo	0.8792	3.1717	0.28590	0.6	1.4	2.3	3.2	4.1	5.0	6.0
15-18 mo	0.8792	3.0649	0.29508	0.6	1.3	2.2	3.1	4.0	4.9	5.9
16-19 mo	0.8792	2.9758	0.30351	0.5	1.2	2.1	3.0	3.9	4.8	5.8
17-20 mo	0.8792	2.9068	0.31089	0.4	1.2	2.0	2.9	3.8	4.8	5.7
18-21 mo	0.8792	2.8507	0.31767	0.4	1.1	2.0	2.9	3.8	4.7	5.7
19-22 mo	0.8792	2.7940	0.32487	0.3	1.1	1.9	2.8	3.7	4.7	5.6
20-23 mo	0.8792	2.7265	0.33332	0.2	1.0	1.8	2.7	3.7	4.6	5.6
21-24 mo	0.8792	2.6405	0.34377	0.2	0.9	1.8	2.6	3.6	4.5	5.5

Table 21 Girls 3-month length increments (cm)

Interval	L	M	S	1st	3rd	5th	15th	25th	50th	75th	85th	95th	97th	99th
0-3 mo	0.8538	10.5967	0.11683	7.8	8.3	8.6	9.3	9.8	10.6	11.4	11.9	12.7	13.0	13.5
1-4 mo	0.8538	8.7743	0.13505	6.1	6.6	6.9	7.6	8.0	8.8	9.6	10.0	10.8	11.0	11.6
2-5 mo	0.8538	7.1455	0.15574	4.6	5.1	5.4	6.0	6.4	7.1	7.9	8.3	9.0	9.3	9.8
3-6 mo	0.8538	5.9428	0.17798	3.6	4.0	4.2	4.9	5.2	5.9	6.7	7.1	7.7	8.0	8.5
4-7 mo	0.8538	5.1554	0.19661	2.9	3.3	3.5	4.1	4.5	5.2	5.8	6.2	6.9	7.1	7.6
5-8 mo	0.8538	4.6834	0.20988	2.5	2.9	3.1	3.7	4.0	4.7	5.4	5.7	6.3	6.6	7.0
6-9 mo	0.8538	4.3922	0.21849	2.3	2.6	2.9	3.4	3.8	4.4	5.0	5.4	6.0	6.2	6.7
7-10 mo	0.8538	4.1971	0.22383	2.1	2.5	2.7	3.2	3.6	4.2	4.8	5.2	5.8	6.0	6.5
8-11 mo	0.8538	4.0329	0.22876	2.0	2.4	2.6	3.1	3.4	4.0	4.7	5.0	5.6	5.8	6.3
9-12 mo	0.8538	3.8692	0.23503	1.9	2.2	2.4	2.9	3.3	3.9	4.5	4.8	5.4	5.6	6.1
10-13 mo	0.8538	3.7174	0.24257	1.7	2.1	2.3	2.8	3.1	3.7	4.3	4.7	5.2	5.5	5.9
11-14 mo	0.8538	3.5892	0.25105	1.6	2.0	2.2	2.7	3.0	3.6	4.2	4.5	5.1	5.3	5.8
12-15 mo	0.8538	3.4811	0.25988	1.5	1.8	2.0	2.6	2.9	3.5	4.1	4.4	5.0	5.2	5.7
13-16 mo	0.8538	3.3844	0.26843	1.4	1.7	1.9	2.5	2.8	3.4	4.0	4.3	4.9	5.1	5.6
14-17 mo	0.8538	3.2934	0.27635	1.3	1.7	1.9	2.4	2.7	3.3	3.9	4.3	4.8	5.1	5.5
15-18 mo	0.8538	3.2051	0.28388	1.2	1.6	1.8	2.3	2.6	3.2	3.8	4.2	4.7	5.0	5.4
16-19 mo	0.8538	3.1173	0.29130	1.1	1.5	1.7	2.2	2.5	3.1	3.7	4.1	4.7	4.9	5.3
17-20 mo	0.8538	3.0295	0.29869	1.1	1.4	1.6	2.1	2.4	3.0	3.6	4.0	4.6	4.8	5.2
18-21 mo	0.8538	2.9427	0.30582	1.0	1.3	1.5	2.0	2.3	2.9	3.6	3.9	4.5	4.7	5.1
19-22 mo	0.8538	2.8576	0.31251	0.9	1.3	1.5	2.0	2.3	2.9	3.5	3.8	4.4	4.6	5.0
20-23 mo	0.8538	2.7779	0.31896	0.9	1.2	1.4	1.9	2.2	2.8	3.4	3.7	4.3	4.5	4.9
21-24 mo	0.8538	2.7091	0.32567	0.8	1.1	1.3	1.8	2.1	2.7	3.3	3.6	4.2	4.4	4.9

Table 21   Girls 3-month length increments (cm) - *continued*

Interval	L	M	S	-3SD	-2SD	-1SD	Median	+1SD	+2SD	+3SD
0-3 mo	0.8538	10.5967	0.11683	7.0	8.2	9.4	10.6	11.8	13.1	14.4
1-4 mo	0.8538	8.7743	0.13505	5.3	6.5	7.6	8.8	10.0	11.2	12.4
2-5 mo	0.8538	7.1455	0.15574	3.9	5.0	6.0	7.1	8.3	9.4	10.6
3-6 mo	0.8538	5.9428	0.17798	2.9	3.9	4.9	5.9	7.0	8.1	9.2
4-7 mo	0.8538	5.1554	0.19661	2.3	3.2	4.2	5.2	6.2	7.2	8.3
5-8 mo	0.8538	4.6834	0.20988	1.9	2.8	3.7	4.7	5.7	6.7	7.8
6-9 mo	0.8538	4.3922	0.21849	1.7	2.5	3.4	4.4	5.4	6.4	7.4
7-10 mo	0.8538	4.1971	0.22383	1.5	2.4	3.3	4.2	5.2	6.1	7.1
8-11 mo	0.8538	4.0329	0.22876	1.4	2.3	3.1	4.0	5.0	5.9	6.9
9-12 mo	0.8538	3.8692	0.23503	1.3	2.1	3.0	3.9	4.8	5.7	6.7
10-13 mo	0.8538	3.7174	0.24257	1.2	2.0	2.8	3.7	4.6	5.6	6.5
11-14 mo	0.8538	3.5892	0.25105	1.1	1.9	2.7	3.6	4.5	5.5	6.4
12-15 mo	0.8538	3.4811	0.25988	1.0	1.8	2.6	3.5	4.4	5.4	6.3
13-16 mo	0.8538	3.3844	0.26843	0.9	1.7	2.5	3.4	4.3	5.3	6.2
14-17 mo	0.8538	3.2934	0.27635	0.8	1.6	2.4	3.3	4.2	5.2	6.2
15-18 mo	0.8538	3.2051	0.28388	0.7	1.5	2.3	3.2	4.1	5.1	6.1
16-19 mo	0.8538	3.1173	0.29130	0.6	1.4	2.2	3.1	4.0	5.0	6.0
17-20 mo	0.8538	3.0295	0.29869	0.6	1.3	2.1	3.0	4.0	4.9	5.9
18-21 mo	0.8538	2.9427	0.30582	0.5	1.2	2.1	2.9	3.9	4.8	5.8
19-22 mo	0.8538	2.8576	0.31251	0.4	1.2	2.0	2.9	3.8	4.7	5.7
20-23 mo	0.8538	2.7779	0.31896	0.4	1.1	1.9	2.8	3.7	4.6	5.6
21-24 mo	0.8538	2.7091	0.32567	0.3	1.0	1.8	2.7	3.6	4.5	5.5

Table 22   Boys 4-month length increments (cm)

Interval	L	M	S	1st	3rd	5th	15th	25th	50th	75th	85th	95th	97th	99th
0-4 mo	1.0138	13.9770	0.10113	10.7	11.3	11.6	12.5	13.0	14.0	14.9	15.4	16.3	16.6	17.3
1-5 mo	1.0138	11.4886	0.12006	8.3	8.9	9.2	10.1	10.6	11.5	12.4	12.9	13.8	14.1	14.7
2-6 mo	1.0138	9.3048	0.13954	6.3	6.9	7.2	8.0	8.4	9.3	10.2	10.6	11.4	11.7	12.3
3-7 mo	1.0138	7.7601	0.15624	4.9	5.5	5.8	6.5	6.9	7.8	8.6	9.0	9.8	10.0	10.6
4-8 mo	1.0138	6.7018	0.16955	4.0	4.6	4.8	5.5	5.9	6.7	7.5	7.9	8.6	8.8	9.3
5-9 mo	1.0138	6.0704	0.17780	3.6	4.0	4.3	5.0	5.3	6.1	6.8	7.2	7.8	8.1	8.6
6-10 mo	1.0138	5.6756	0.18311	3.2	3.7	4.0	4.6	5.0	5.7	6.4	6.8	7.4	7.6	8.1
7-11 mo	1.0138	5.3939	0.18754	3.0	3.5	3.7	4.3	4.7	5.4	6.1	6.4	7.1	7.3	7.7
8-12 mo	1.0138	5.1699	0.19138	2.9	3.3	3.5	4.1	4.5	5.2	5.8	6.2	6.8	7.0	7.5
9-13 mo	1.0138	4.9623	0.19512	2.7	3.1	3.4	4.0	4.3	5.0	5.6	6.0	6.6	6.8	7.2
10-14 mo	1.0138	4.7773	0.19880	2.6	3.0	3.2	3.8	4.1	4.8	5.4	5.8	6.3	6.6	7.0
11-15 mo	1.0138	4.6014	0.20286	2.4	2.8	3.1	3.6	4.0	4.6	5.2	5.6	6.1	6.4	6.8
12-16 mo	1.0138	4.4487	0.20707	2.3	2.7	2.9	3.5	3.8	4.4	5.1	5.4	6.0	6.2	6.6
13-17 mo	1.0138	4.3123	0.21158	2.2	2.6	2.8	3.4	3.7	4.3	4.9	5.3	5.8	6.0	6.4
14-18 mo	1.0138	4.1833	0.21644	2.1	2.5	2.7	3.2	3.6	4.2	4.8	5.1	5.7	5.9	6.3
15-19 mo	1.0138	4.0680	0.22124	2.0	2.4	2.6	3.1	3.5	4.1	4.7	5.0	5.5	5.8	6.2
16-20 mo	1.0138	3.9584	0.22619	1.9	2.3	2.5	3.0	3.4	4.0	4.6	4.9	5.4	5.6	6.0
17-21 mo	1.0138	3.8600	0.23092	1.8	2.2	2.4	2.9	3.3	3.9	4.5	4.8	5.3	5.5	5.9
18-22 mo	1.0138	3.7663	0.23577	1.7	2.1	2.3	2.8	3.2	3.8	4.4	4.7	5.2	5.4	5.8
19-23 mo	1.0138	3.6815	0.24063	1.6	2.0	2.2	2.8	3.1	3.7	4.3	4.6	5.1	5.3	5.7
20-24 mo	1.0138	3.6058	0.24530	1.5	1.9	2.1	2.7	3.0	3.6	4.2	4.5	5.1	5.3	5.7

Table 22 Boys 4-month length increments (cm) - *continued*

Interval	L	M	S	-3SD	-2SD	-1SD	Median	+1SD	+2SD	+3SD
0-4 mo	1.0138	13.9770	0.10113	9.7	11.1	12.6	14.0	15.4	16.8	18.2
1-5 mo	1.0138	11.4886	0.12006	7.3	8.7	10.1	11.5	12.9	14.2	15.6
2-6 mo	1.0138	9.3048	0.13954	5.4	6.7	8.0	9.3	10.6	11.9	13.2
3-7 mo	1.0138	7.7601	0.15624	4.1	5.3	6.5	7.8	9.0	10.2	11.4
4-8 mo	1.0138	6.7018	0.16955	3.3	4.4	5.6	6.7	7.8	9.0	10.1
5-9 mo	1.0138	6.0704	0.17780	2.8	3.9	5.0	6.1	7.1	8.2	9.3
6-10 mo	1.0138	5.6756	0.18311	2.5	3.6	4.6	5.7	6.7	7.7	8.8
7-11 mo	1.0138	5.3939	0.18754	2.3	3.4	4.4	5.4	6.4	7.4	8.4
8-12 mo	1.0138	5.1699	0.19138	2.2	3.2	4.2	5.2	6.2	7.1	8.1
9-13 mo	1.0138	4.9623	0.19512	2.0	3.0	4.0	5.0	5.9	6.9	7.9
10-14 mo	1.0138	4.7773	0.19880	1.9	2.9	3.8	4.8	5.7	6.7	7.6
11-15 mo	1.0138	4.6014	0.20286	1.8	2.7	3.7	4.6	5.5	6.5	7.4
12-16 mo	1.0138	4.4487	0.20707	1.7	2.6	3.5	4.4	5.4	6.3	7.2
13-17 mo	1.0138	4.3123	0.21158	1.6	2.5	3.4	4.3	5.2	6.1	7.0
14-18 mo	1.0138	4.1833	0.21644	1.5	2.4	3.3	4.2	5.1	6.0	6.9
15-19 mo	1.0138	4.0680	0.22124	1.4	2.3	3.2	4.1	5.0	5.9	6.8
16-20 mo	1.0138	3.9584	0.22619	1.3	2.2	3.1	4.0	4.9	5.7	6.6
17-21 mo	1.0138	3.8600	0.23092	1.2	2.1	3.0	3.9	4.8	5.6	6.5
18-22 mo	1.0138	3.7663	0.23577	1.1	2.0	2.9	3.8	4.7	5.5	6.4
19-23 mo	1.0138	3.6815	0.24063	1.0	1.9	2.8	3.7	4.6	5.4	6.3
20-24 mo	1.0138	3.6058	0.24530	0.9	1.8	2.7	3.6	4.5	5.4	6.2

Table 23   Girls 4-month length increments (cm)

Interval	L	M	S	1st	3rd	5th	15th	25th	50th	75th	85th	95th	97th	99th
0-4 mo	0.8123	13.0081	0.10744	9.8	10.4	10.7	11.6	12.1	13.0	14.0	14.5	15.3	15.7	16.3
1-5 mo	0.8123	10.6621	0.12126	7.7	8.3	8.6	9.3	9.8	10.7	11.5	12.0	12.8	13.1	13.7
2-6 mo	0.8123	8.7302	0.13625	6.1	6.5	6.8	7.5	7.9	8.7	9.5	10.0	10.7	11.0	11.6
3-7 mo	0.8123	7.4606	0.15069	4.9	5.4	5.7	6.3	6.7	7.5	8.2	8.6	9.4	9.6	10.2
4-8 mo	0.8123	6.5992	0.16368	4.2	4.6	4.9	5.5	5.9	6.6	7.3	7.7	8.4	8.7	9.2
5-9 mo	0.8123	6.0664	0.17240	3.7	4.2	4.4	5.0	5.4	6.1	6.8	7.2	7.8	8.1	8.6
6-10 mo	0.8123	5.7273	0.17782	3.5	3.9	4.1	4.7	5.0	5.7	6.4	6.8	7.4	7.7	8.2
7-11 mo	0.8123	5.4731	0.18189	3.3	3.7	3.9	4.5	4.8	5.5	6.2	6.5	7.2	7.4	7.9
8-12 mo	0.8123	5.2575	0.18562	3.1	3.5	3.7	4.3	4.6	5.3	5.9	6.3	6.9	7.1	7.6
9-13 mo	0.8123	5.0550	0.18974	2.9	3.3	3.5	4.1	4.4	5.1	5.7	6.1	6.7	6.9	7.4
10-14 mo	0.8123	4.8763	0.19407	2.8	3.2	3.4	3.9	4.2	4.9	5.5	5.9	6.5	6.7	7.2
11-15 mo	0.8123	4.7084	0.19893	2.6	3.0	3.2	3.8	4.1	4.7	5.3	5.7	6.3	6.5	7.0
12-16 mo	0.8123	4.5658	0.20385	2.5	2.9	3.1	3.6	3.9	4.6	5.2	5.5	6.1	6.4	6.8
13-17 mo	0.8123	4.4427	0.20880	2.4	2.8	3.0	3.5	3.8	4.4	5.1	5.4	6.0	6.2	6.7
14-18 mo	0.8123	4.3256	0.21372	2.3	2.7	2.9	3.4	3.7	4.3	5.0	5.3	5.9	6.1	6.6
15-19 mo	0.8123	4.2141	0.21816	2.2	2.6	2.8	3.3	3.6	4.2	4.8	5.2	5.8	6.0	6.4
16-20 mo	0.8123	4.0974	0.22240	2.1	2.5	2.7	3.2	3.5	4.1	4.7	5.1	5.6	5.9	6.3
17-21 mo	0.8123	3.9825	0.22623	2.0	2.4	2.6	3.1	3.4	4.0	4.6	4.9	5.5	5.7	6.2
18-22 mo	0.8123	3.8660	0.22998	1.9	2.3	2.5	3.0	3.3	3.9	4.5	4.8	5.4	5.6	6.0
19-23 mo	0.8123	3.7559	0.23357	1.8	2.2	2.4	2.9	3.2	3.8	4.4	4.7	5.2	5.5	5.9
20-24 mo	0.8123	3.6558	0.23694	1.8	2.1	2.3	2.8	3.1	3.7	4.2	4.6	5.1	5.3	5.8

Table 23   Girls 4-month length increments (cm) – *continued*

Interval	L	M	S	-3SD	-2SD	-1SD	Median	+1SD	+2SD	+3SD
0-4 mo	0.8123	13.0081	0.10744	9.0	10.3	11.6	13.0	14.4	15.9	17.3
1-5 mo	0.8123	10.6621	0.12126	6.9	8.1	9.4	10.7	12.0	13.3	14.7
2-6 mo	0.8123	8.7302	0.13625	5.3	6.4	7.6	8.7	9.9	11.2	12.4
3-7 mo	0.8123	7.4606	0.15069	4.2	5.3	6.4	7.5	8.6	9.8	11.0
4-8 mo	0.8123	6.5992	0.16368	3.5	4.5	5.5	6.6	7.7	8.8	10.0
5-9 mo	0.8123	6.0664	0.17240	3.1	4.0	5.0	6.1	7.1	8.2	9.3
6-10 mo	0.8123	5.7273	0.17782	2.8	3.8	4.7	5.7	6.8	7.8	8.9
7-11 mo	0.8123	5.4731	0.18189	2.7	3.6	4.5	5.5	6.5	7.5	8.6
8-12 mo	0.8123	5.2575	0.18562	2.5	3.4	4.3	5.3	6.2	7.3	8.3
9-13 mo	0.8123	5.0550	0.18974	2.4	3.2	4.1	5.1	6.0	7.0	8.1
10-14 mo	0.8123	4.8763	0.19407	2.2	3.1	3.9	4.9	5.8	6.8	7.9
11-15 mo	0.8123	4.7084	0.19893	2.1	2.9	3.8	4.7	5.7	6.6	7.7
12-16 mo	0.8123	4.5658	0.20385	2.0	2.8	3.7	4.6	5.5	6.5	7.5
13-17 mo	0.8123	4.4427	0.20880	1.9	2.7	3.5	4.4	5.4	6.4	7.4
14-18 mo	0.8123	4.3256	0.21372	1.7	2.6	3.4	4.3	5.3	6.2	7.2
15-19 mo	0.8123	4.2141	0.21816	1.7	2.5	3.3	4.2	5.2	6.1	7.1
16-20 mo	0.8123	4.0974	0.22240	1.6	2.4	3.2	4.1	5.0	6.0	7.0
17-21 mo	0.8123	3.9825	0.22623	1.5	2.3	3.1	4.0	4.9	5.9	6.8
18-22 mo	0.8123	3.8660	0.22998	1.4	2.2	3.0	3.9	4.8	5.7	6.7
19-23 mo	0.8123	3.7559	0.23357	1.3	2.1	2.9	3.8	4.7	5.6	6.5
20-24 mo	0.8123	3.6558	0.23694	1.3	2.0	2.8	3.7	4.5	5.5	6.4

Table 24 Boys 6-month length increments (cm)

Interval	L	M	S	1st	3rd	5th	15th	25th	50th	75th	85th	95th	97th	99th
0-6 mo	0.9027	17.6547	0.09452	13.8	14.5	14.9	15.9	16.5	17.7	18.8	19.4	20.4	20.8	21.6
1-7 mo	0.9027	14.7110	0.10935	11.0	11.7	12.1	13.1	13.6	14.7	15.8	16.4	17.4	17.8	18.5
2-8 mo	0.9027	12.3097	0.12383	8.8	9.5	9.8	10.7	11.3	12.3	13.3	13.9	14.8	15.2	15.9
3-9 mo	0.9027	10.5768	0.13570	7.3	7.9	8.2	9.1	9.6	10.6	11.5	12.1	13.0	13.3	14.0
4-10 mo	0.9027	9.4000	0.14407	6.3	6.9	7.2	8.0	8.5	9.4	10.3	10.8	11.7	12.0	12.6
5-11 mo	0.9027	8.6282	0.14919	5.7	6.2	6.5	7.3	7.8	8.6	9.5	10.0	10.8	11.1	11.7
6-12 mo	0.9027	8.1114	0.15162	5.3	5.8	6.1	6.8	7.3	8.1	8.9	9.4	10.2	10.5	11.0
7-13 mo	0.9027	7.7366	0.15255	5.0	5.6	5.8	6.5	6.9	7.7	8.5	9.0	9.7	10.0	10.5
8-14 mo	0.9027	7.4335	0.15299	4.8	5.3	5.6	6.3	6.7	7.4	8.2	8.6	9.3	9.6	10.1
9-15 mo	0.9027	7.1621	0.15364	4.7	5.1	5.4	6.0	6.4	7.2	7.9	8.3	9.0	9.3	9.8
10-16 mo	0.9027	6.9165	0.15479	4.5	4.9	5.2	5.8	6.2	6.9	7.6	8.0	8.7	9.0	9.4
11-17 mo	0.9027	6.6927	0.15649	4.3	4.8	5.0	5.6	6.0	6.7	7.4	7.8	8.4	8.7	9.2
12-18 mo	0.9027	6.4830	0.15863	4.1	4.6	4.8	5.4	5.8	6.5	7.2	7.6	8.2	8.4	8.9
13-19 mo	0.9027	6.2862	0.16108	4.0	4.4	4.6	5.2	5.6	6.3	7.0	7.3	8.0	8.2	8.7
14-20 mo	0.9027	6.1061	0.16362	3.8	4.3	4.5	5.1	5.4	6.1	6.8	7.1	7.8	8.0	8.5
15-21 mo	0.9027	5.9431	0.16610	3.7	4.1	4.3	4.9	5.3	5.9	6.6	7.0	7.6	7.8	8.3
16-22 mo	0.9027	5.7899	0.16861	3.6	4.0	4.2	4.8	5.1	5.8	6.5	6.8	7.4	7.7	8.1
17-23 mo	0.9027	5.6425	0.17124	3.4	3.9	4.1	4.7	5.0	5.6	6.3	6.7	7.3	7.5	7.9
18-24 mo	0.9027	5.5018	0.17392	3.3	3.7	4.0	4.5	4.9	5.5	6.2	6.5	7.1	7.3	7.8

Table 24 Boys 6-month length increments (cm) - *continued*

Interval	L	M	S	-3SD	-2SD	-1SD	Median	+1SD	+2SD	+3SD
0-6 mo	0.9027	17.6547	0.09452	12.7	14.3	16.0	17.7	19.3	21.0	22.7
1-7 mo	0.9027	14.7110	0.10935	10.0	11.5	13.1	14.7	16.3	18.0	19.6
2-8 mo	0.9027	12.3097	0.12383	7.8	9.3	10.8	12.3	13.8	15.4	17.0
3-9 mo	0.9027	10.5768	0.13570	6.4	7.7	9.2	10.6	12.0	13.5	15.0
4-10 mo	0.9027	9.4000	0.14407	5.4	6.7	8.1	9.4	10.8	12.1	13.5
5-11 mo	0.9027	8.6282	0.14919	4.9	6.1	7.4	8.6	9.9	11.2	12.6
6-12 mo	0.9027	8.1114	0.15162	4.5	5.7	6.9	8.1	9.3	10.6	11.9
7-13 mo	0.9027	7.7366	0.15255	4.3	5.4	6.6	7.7	8.9	10.1	11.3
8-14 mo	0.9027	7.4335	0.15299	4.1	5.2	6.3	7.4	8.6	9.7	10.9
9-15 mo	0.9027	7.1621	0.15364	3.9	5.0	6.1	7.2	8.3	9.4	10.5
10-16 mo	0.9027	6.9165	0.15479	3.8	4.8	5.9	6.9	8.0	9.1	10.2
11-17 mo	0.9027	6.6927	0.15649	3.6	4.6	5.7	6.7	7.7	8.8	9.9
12-18 mo	0.9027	6.4830	0.15863	3.5	4.5	5.5	6.5	7.5	8.6	9.6
13-19 mo	0.9027	6.2862	0.16108	3.3	4.3	5.3	6.3	7.3	8.3	9.4
14-20 mo	0.9027	6.1061	0.16362	3.2	4.1	5.1	6.1	7.1	8.1	9.2
15-21 mo	0.9027	5.9431	0.16610	3.1	4.0	5.0	5.9	6.9	7.9	9.0
16-22 mo	0.9027	5.7899	0.16861	2.9	3.9	4.8	5.8	6.8	7.8	8.8
17-23 mo	0.9027	5.6425	0.17124	2.8	3.7	4.7	5.6	6.6	7.6	8.6
18-24 mo	0.9027	5.5018	0.17392	2.7	3.6	4.6	5.5	6.5	7.4	8.4

Table 25 Girls 6-month length increments (cm)

Interval	L	M	S	1st	3rd	5th	15th	25th	50th	75th	85th	95th	97th	99th
0-6 mo	0.7138	16.4915	0.09904	12.8	13.5	13.9	14.8	15.4	16.5	17.6	18.2	19.2	19.6	20.4
1-7 mo	0.7138	13.8733	0.10884	10.5	11.1	11.5	12.3	12.9	13.9	14.9	15.5	16.4	16.8	17.5
2-8 mo	0.7138	11.8137	0.11821	8.7	9.3	9.6	10.4	10.9	11.8	12.8	13.3	14.2	14.5	15.2
3-9 mo	0.7138	10.3499	0.12639	7.4	8.0	8.3	9.0	9.5	10.3	11.2	11.7	12.6	12.9	13.5
4-10 mo	0.7138	9.3426	0.13290	6.6	7.1	7.4	8.1	8.5	9.3	10.2	10.7	11.4	11.8	12.4
5-11 mo	0.7138	8.6770	0.13782	6.0	6.5	6.8	7.5	7.9	8.7	9.5	9.9	10.7	11.0	11.6
6-12 mo	0.7138	8.2244	0.14171	5.6	6.1	6.4	7.0	7.4	8.2	9.0	9.5	10.2	10.5	11.1
7-13 mo	0.7138	7.8787	0.14512	5.4	5.8	6.1	6.7	7.1	7.9	8.7	9.1	9.8	10.1	10.7
8-14 mo	0.7138	7.5879	0.14836	5.1	5.6	5.8	6.4	6.8	7.6	8.4	8.8	9.5	9.8	10.3
9-15 mo	0.7138	7.3259	0.15166	4.9	5.3	5.6	6.2	6.6	7.3	8.1	8.5	9.2	9.5	10.0
10-16 mo	0.7138	7.0897	0.15514	4.7	5.1	5.3	6.0	6.4	7.1	7.8	8.3	9.0	9.2	9.8
11-17 mo	0.7138	6.8778	0.15880	4.5	4.9	5.2	5.8	6.2	6.9	7.6	8.0	8.7	9.0	9.5
12-18 mo	0.7138	6.6823	0.16252	4.3	4.7	5.0	5.6	6.0	6.7	7.4	7.8	8.5	8.8	9.3
13-19 mo	0.7138	6.4984	0.16617	4.1	4.6	4.8	5.4	5.8	6.5	7.2	7.6	8.3	8.6	9.1
14-20 mo	0.7138	6.3217	0.16964	4.0	4.4	4.6	5.2	5.6	6.3	7.1	7.5	8.2	8.4	9.0
15-21 mo	0.7138	6.1484	0.17287	3.8	4.2	4.5	5.1	5.4	6.1	6.9	7.3	8.0	8.2	8.8
16-22 mo	0.7138	5.9770	0.17591	3.7	4.1	4.3	4.9	5.3	6.0	6.7	7.1	7.8	8.0	8.6
17-23 mo	0.7138	5.8083	0.17884	3.5	4.0	4.2	4.8	5.1	5.8	6.5	6.9	7.6	7.9	8.4
18-24 mo	0.7138	5.6454	0.18169	3.4	3.8	4.0	4.6	5.0	5.6	6.3	6.7	7.4	7.7	8.2

Table 25 Girls 6-month length increments (cm) - *continued*

Interval	L	M	S	-3SD	-2SD	-1SD	Median	+1SD	+2SD	+3SD
0-6 mo	0.7138	16.4915	0.09904	11.8	13.3	14.9	16.5	18.1	19.8	21.6
1-7 mo	0.7138	13.8733	0.10884	9.6	11.0	12.4	13.9	15.4	17.0	18.6
2-8 mo	0.7138	11.8137	0.11821	7.8	9.1	10.4	11.8	13.2	14.7	16.2
3-9 mo	0.7138	10.3499	0.12639	6.7	7.8	9.1	10.3	11.7	13.1	14.5
4-10 mo	0.7138	9.3426	0.13290	5.8	7.0	8.1	9.3	10.6	11.9	13.3
5-11 mo	0.7138	8.6770	0.13782	5.3	6.4	7.5	8.7	9.9	11.2	12.5
6-12 mo	0.7138	8.2244	0.14171	5.0	6.0	7.1	8.2	9.4	10.6	11.9
7-13 mo	0.7138	7.8787	0.14512	4.7	5.7	6.8	7.9	9.0	10.3	11.5
8-14 mo	0.7138	7.5879	0.14836	4.4	5.4	6.5	7.6	8.7	9.9	11.2
9-15 mo	0.7138	7.3259	0.15166	4.2	5.2	6.2	7.3	8.5	9.6	10.9
10-16 mo	0.7138	7.0897	0.15514	4.0	5.0	6.0	7.1	8.2	9.4	10.6
11-17 mo	0.7138	6.8778	0.15880	3.8	4.8	5.8	6.9	8.0	9.2	10.4
12-18 mo	0.7138	6.6823	0.16252	3.7	4.6	5.6	6.7	7.8	9.0	10.2
13-19 mo	0.7138	6.4984	0.16617	3.5	4.4	5.4	6.5	7.6	8.8	10.0
14-20 mo	0.7138	6.3217	0.16964	3.4	4.3	5.3	6.3	7.4	8.6	9.8
15-21 mo	0.7138	6.1484	0.17287	3.2	4.1	5.1	6.1	7.2	8.4	9.6
16-22 mo	0.7138	5.9770	0.17591	3.1	4.0	5.0	6.0	7.1	8.2	9.4
17-23 mo	0.7138	5.8083	0.17884	3.0	3.8	4.8	5.8	6.9	8.0	9.1
18-24 mo	0.7138	5.6454	0.18169	2.8	3.7	4.6	5.6	6.7	7.8	8.9

Appendix A4 Diagnostics

A4.1a 2-month intervals for boys

Table A4.1   Q-test for z-scores from selected model [BCPE(x=age$^{0.05}$, df(μ)=9, df(σ)=7, df(v)=1, τ=2)] for 2-month length velocity for boys

Age (days)	Group	N	z1	z2	z3
55 to 76	**0-2 mo**	422	-0.4	0.6	-1.9
76 to 107	**1-3 mo**	417	1.5	-1.3	2.1
107 to 137	**2-4 mo**	416	-0.9	0.3	1.1
137 to 168	**3-5 mo**	413	0.7	-0.1	1.6
168 to 198	**4-6 mo**	416	-0.8	0.3	0.5
198 to 229	**5-7 mo**	412	-0.6	0.9	0.3
229 to 259	**6-8 mo**	417	-0.4	-0.5	-1.1
259 to 289	**7-9 mo**	409	0.0	1.1	0.4
289 to 320	**8-10 mo**	404	0.8	-0.7	-1.9
320 to 350	**9-11 mo**	411	0.4	0.8	-0.1
350 to 396	**10-12 mo**	405	-0.6	-1.8	-0.6
396 to 457	**12-14 mo**	415	0.6	1.0	0.4
457 to 518	**14-16 mo**	410	-1.0	0.7	-1.0
518 to 579	**16-18 mo**	407	0.8	-1.0	-2.7
579 to 640	**18-20 mo**	412	-0.9	0.9	1.0
640 to 701	**20-22 mo**	415	0.9	0.0	-1.0
701 to 738	**22-24 mo**	414	-0.8	1.2	-2.0
Overall Q stats		7015	10.0	13.3	31.8
degrees of freedom			8.0	13.0	16.0
p-value			0.2625	0.4241	0.0105

Note: Absolute values of z1, z2 or z3 larger than 2 indicate misfit of, respectively, mean, variance or skewness.

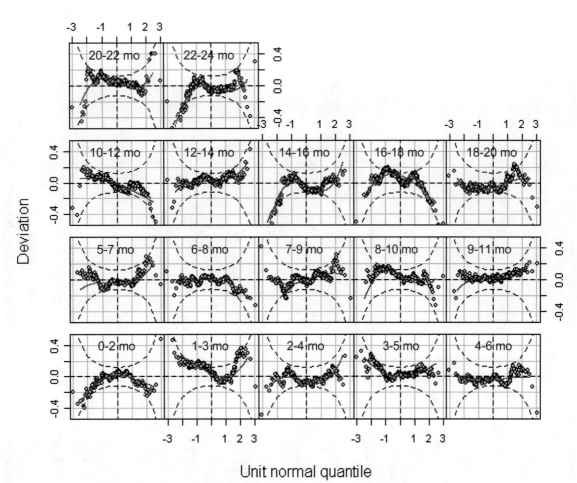

Unit normal quantile

Figure A4.1 Worm plots from selected model [BCPE(x=age$^{0.05}$, df(μ)=9, df(σ)=7, df(ν)=1, τ=2)] for 2-month length velocity for boys

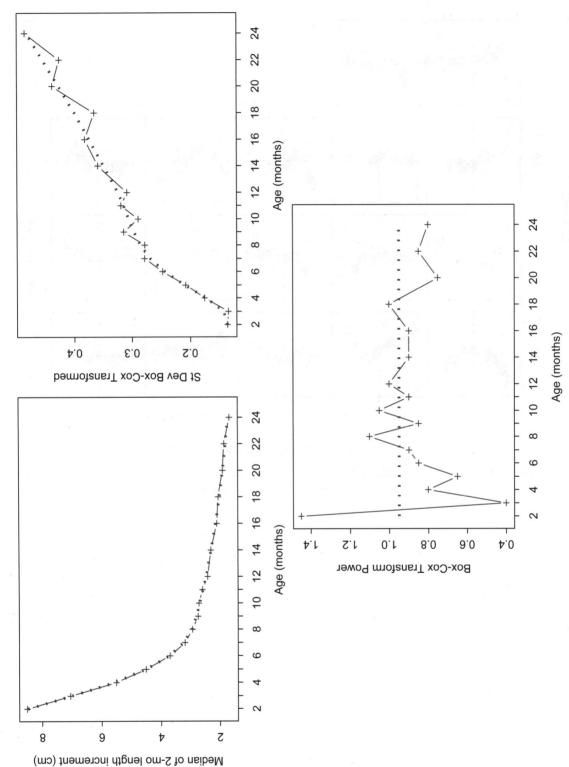

Figure A4.2 Fitting of the μ, σ, and ν curves of selected model for 2-month length velocity for boys

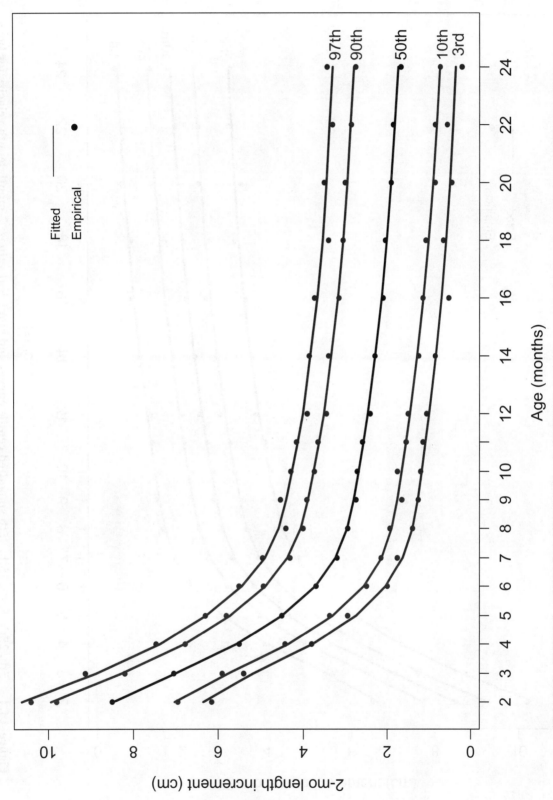

Figure A4.3   3rd, 10th, 50th, 90th, 97th smoothed centile curves and empirical values: 2-month length velocity for boys

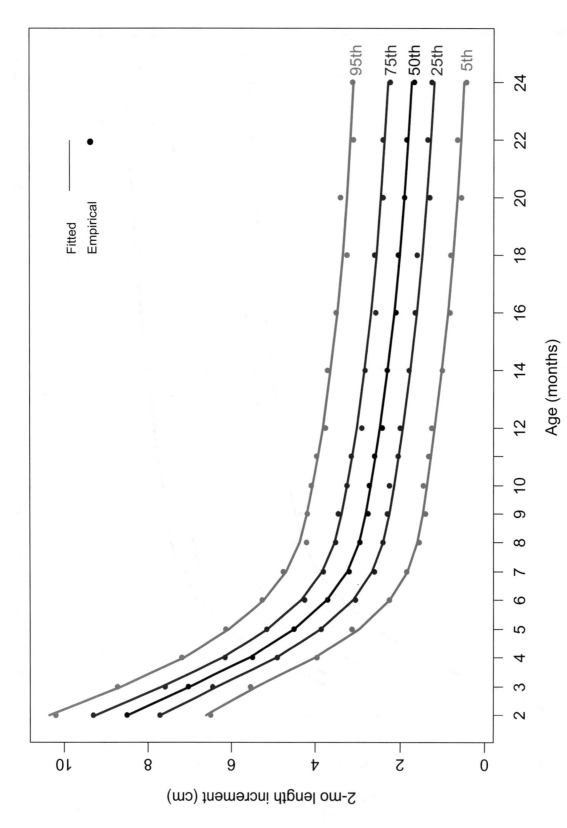

Figure A4.4   5th, 25th, 50th, 75th, 95th smoothed centile curves and empirical values: 2-month length velocity for boys

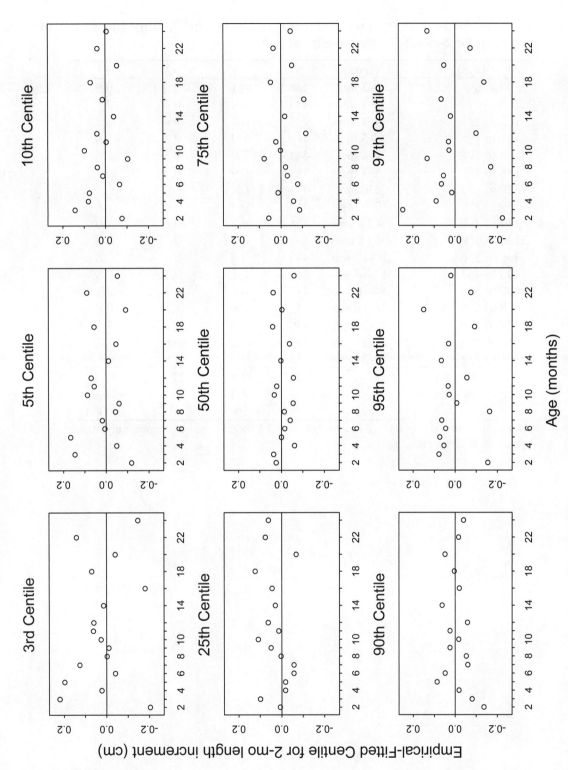

Figure A4.5 Centile residuals from fitting selected model for 2-month length velocity for boys

A4.1b 2-month intervals for girls

Table A4.2   Q-test for z-scores from selected model [BCPE(x=age$^{0.05}$, df(μ)=10, df(σ)=7, df(v)=1, τ=2)] for 2-month length velocity for girls

Age (days)	Group	N	z1	z2	z3
58 to 76	**0-2 mo**	446	0.1	0.5	0.9
76 to 107	**1-3 mo**	443	0.4	-0.7	2.5
107 to 137	**2-4 mo**	441	-0.7	-0.4	-1.2
137 to 168	**3-5 mo**	445	1.2	0.3	-1.6
168 to 198	**4-6 mo**	441	-0.9	0.8	1.0
198 to 229	**5-7 mo**	444	-0.9	-0.9	-0.7
229 to 259	**6-8 mo**	441	0.4	0.0	-0.8
259 to 289	**7-9 mo**	444	0.4	2.0	1.8
289 to 320	**8-10 mo**	438	-0.4	-0.6	-1.0
320 to 350	**9-11 mo**	437	0.1	-0.7	0.6
350 to 396	**10-12 mo**	444	0.4	-0.6	-0.8
396 to 457	**12-14 mo**	449	0.1	0.7	-0.8
457 to 518	**14-16 mo**	442	-0.9	0.2	-2.3
518 to 579	**16-18 mo**	442	0.6	1.6	-0.8
579 to 640	**18-20 mo**	439	-0.5	0.4	-3.3
640 to 701	**20-22 mo**	433	-0.2	0.8	-2.4
701 to 738	**22-24 mo**	435	-0.3	0.8	-0.6
Overall Q stats		7504	5.8	12.1	42.1
degrees of freedom			7.0	13.0	16.0
p-value			0.5606	0.5170	0.0004

Note: Absolute values of z1, z2 or z3 larger than 2 indicate misfit of, respectively, mean, variance or skewness.

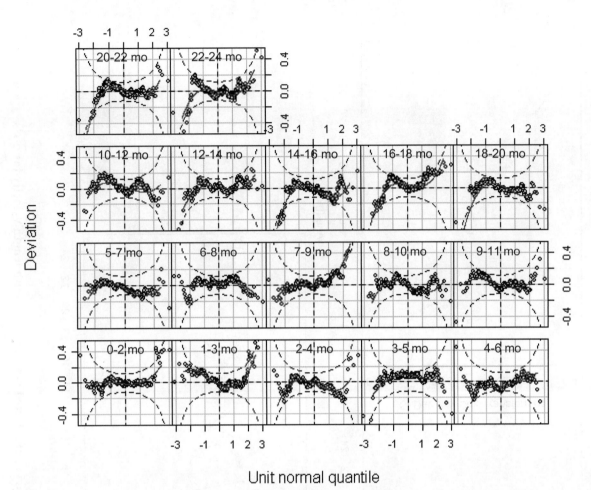

Unit normal quantile

Figure A4.6 Worm plots from selected model [BCPE(x=age$^{0.05}$, df(μ)=10, df(σ)=7, df(ν)=1, τ=2)] for 2-month length velocity for girls

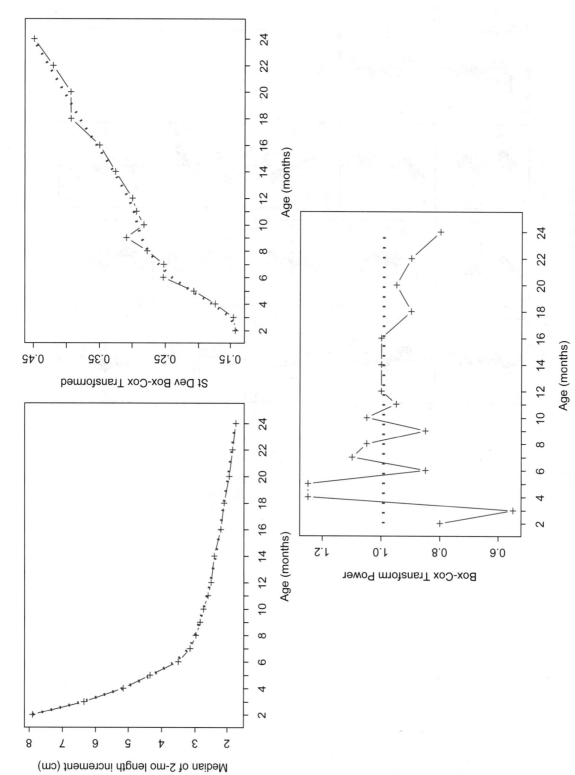

Figure A4.7 Fitting of the μ, σ, and ν curves of selected model for 2-month length velocity for girls

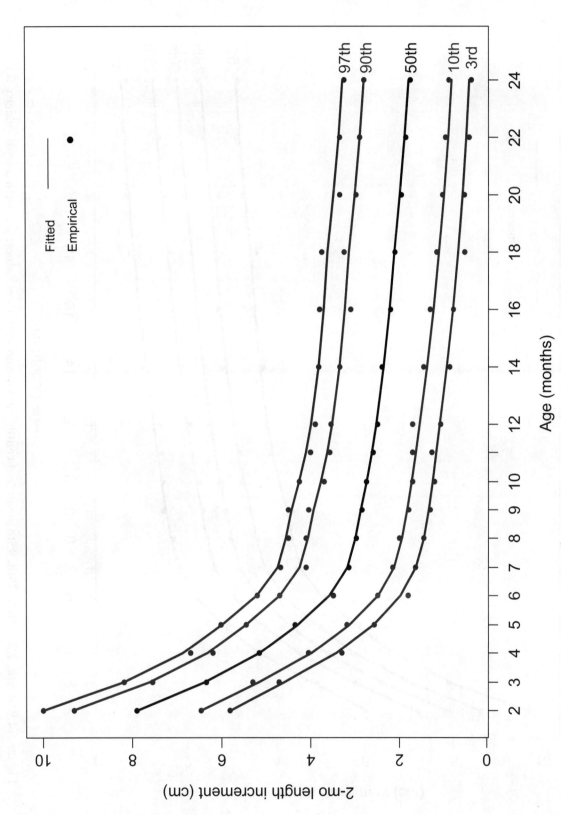

Figure A4.8   3rd, 10th, 50th, 90th, 97th smoothed centile curves and empirical values: 2-month length velocity for girls

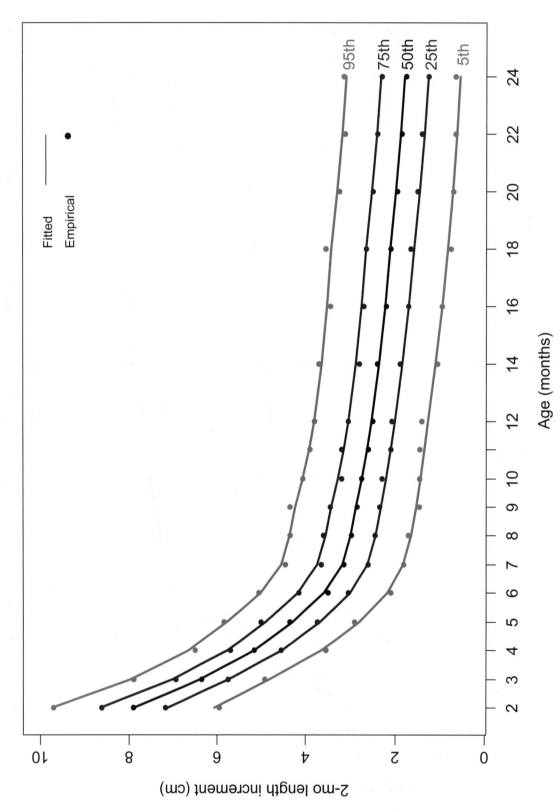

Figure A4.9   5th, 25th, 50th, 75th, 95th smoothed centile curves and empirical values: 2-month length velocity for girls

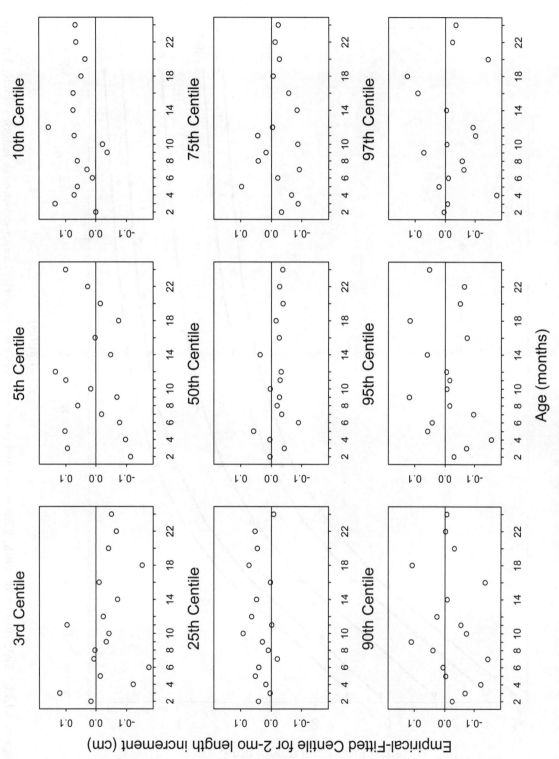

Figure A4.10 Centile residuals from fitting selected model for 2-month length velocity for girls

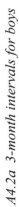

A4.2a 3-month intervals for boys

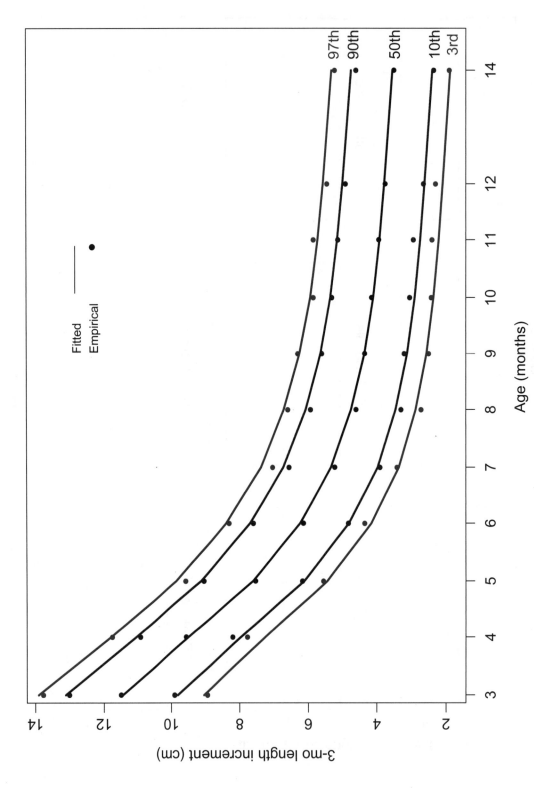

Figure A4.11   3rd, 10th, 50th, 90th, 97th smoothed centile curves and empirical values: 3-month length velocity for boys

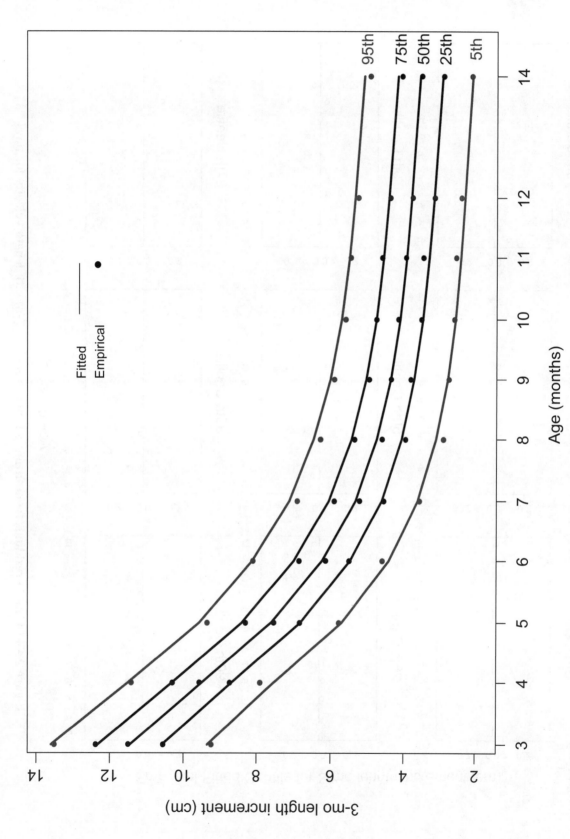

Figure A4.12 5th, 25th, 50th, 75th, 95th smoothed centile curves and empirical values: 3-month length velocity for boys

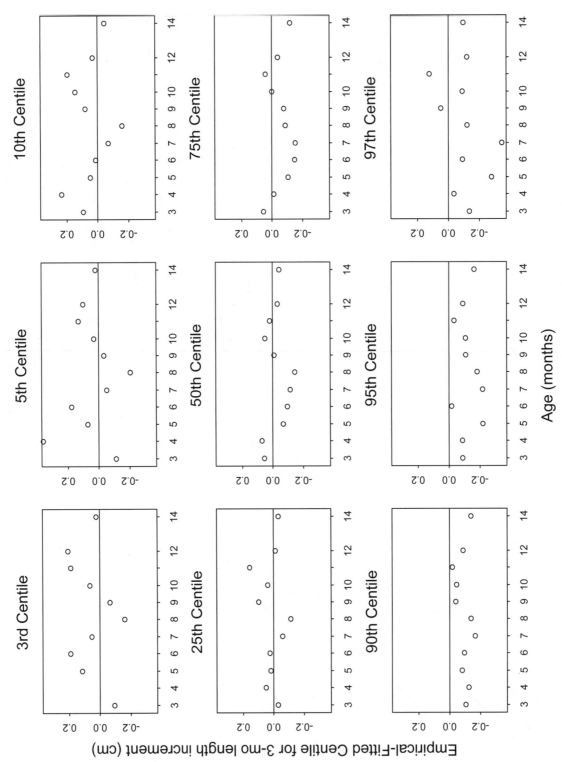

Figure A4.13 Centile residuals from fitting selected model for 3-month length velocity for boys

A4.2b 3-month intervals for girls

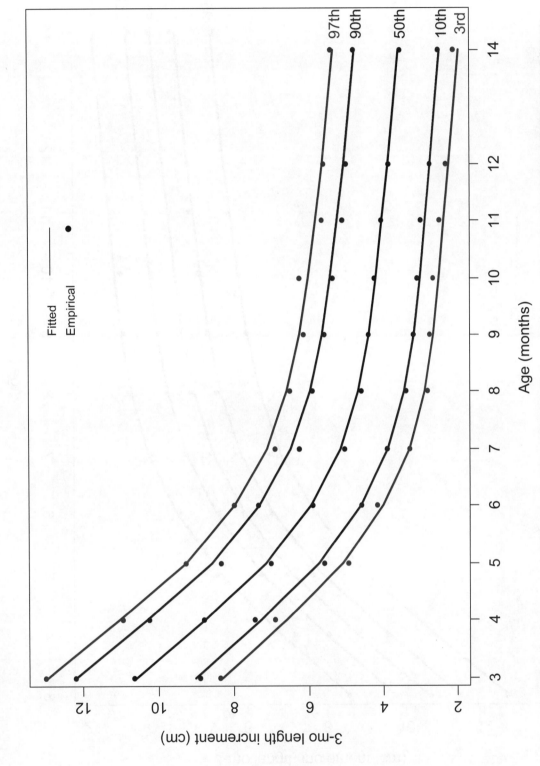

Figure A4.14 3rd, 10th, 50th, 90th, 97th smoothed centile curves and empirical values: 3-month length velocity for girls

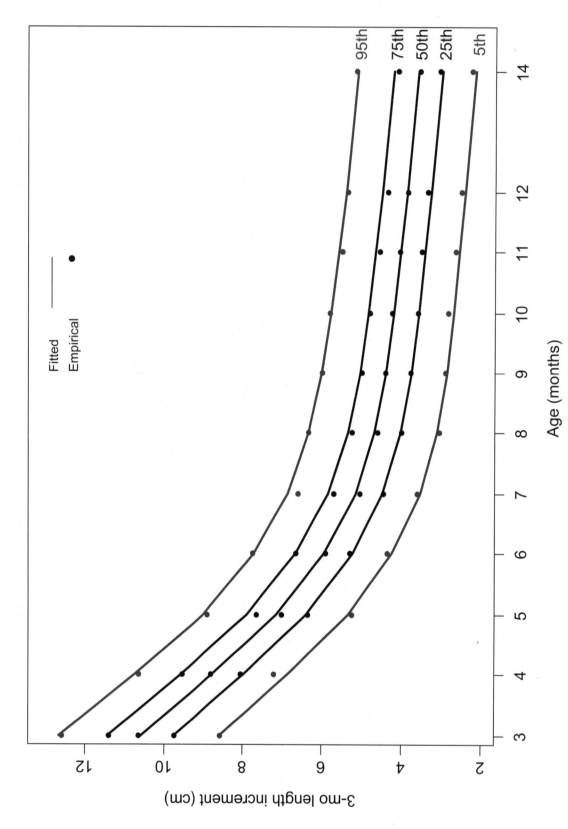

Figure A4.15   5th, 25th, 50th, 75th, 95th smoothed centile curves and empirical values: 3-month length velocity for girls

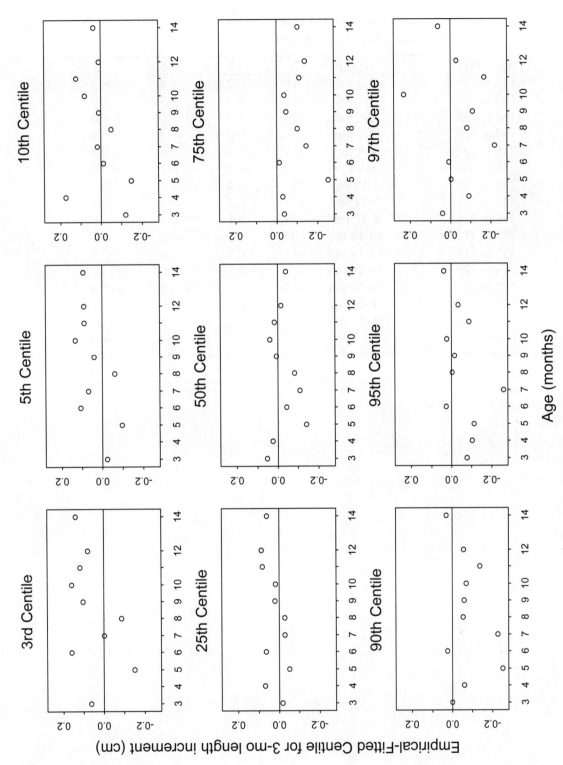

Figure A4.16 Centile residuals from fitting selected model for 3-month length velocity for girls

A4.3a 4-month intervals for boys

Table A4.3 **Q-test for z-scores from selected model [BCPE(x=age$^{0.05}$, df(μ)=8, df(σ)=5, df(ν)=1, τ=2)] for 4-month length velocity for boys**

Age (days)	Group	N	z1	z2	z3
113 to 137	**0-4 mo**	418	-0.2	0.4	-0.2
137 to 168	**1-5 mo**	416	2.2	-1.3	1.9
168 to 198	**2-6 mo**	420	-1.2	0.0	1.4
198 to 229	**3-7 mo**	413	0.0	-0.3	0.9
229 to 259	**4-8 mo**	411	-1.4	1.8	0.3
259 to 289	**5-9 mo**	408	-0.5	0.8	0.0
289 to 320	**6-10 mo**	407	0.4	-1.5	-2.2
320 to 350	**7-11 mo**	413	0.7	-0.2	-0.3
350 to 396	**8-12 mo**	415	-0.1	0.4	1.9
396 to 457	**10-14 mo**	402	0.3	-0.2	-0.2
457 to 518	**12-16 mo**	413	0.0	-0.6	-0.2
518 to 579	**14-18 mo**	409	0.1	0.0	-0.4
579 to 640	**16-20 mo**	413	-0.1	0.9	-0.8
640 to 701	**18-22 mo**	408	-0.1	-0.9	2.1
701 to 750	**20-24 mo**	417	-0.1	0.5	-0.5
Overall Q stats		6183	9.1	10.5	20.4
degrees of freedom			7.0	12.0	14.0
p-value			0.2463	0.5688	0.1184

Note: Absolute values of z1, z2 or z3 larger than 2 indicate misfit of, respectively, mean, variance or skewness.

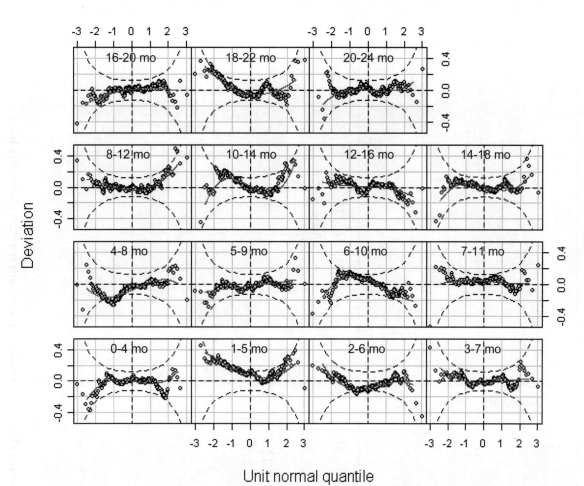

Figure A4.17 Worm plots from selected model [BCPE(x=age$^{0.05}$, df(μ)=8, df(σ)=5, df(ν)=1, τ=2)] for 4-month length velocity for boys

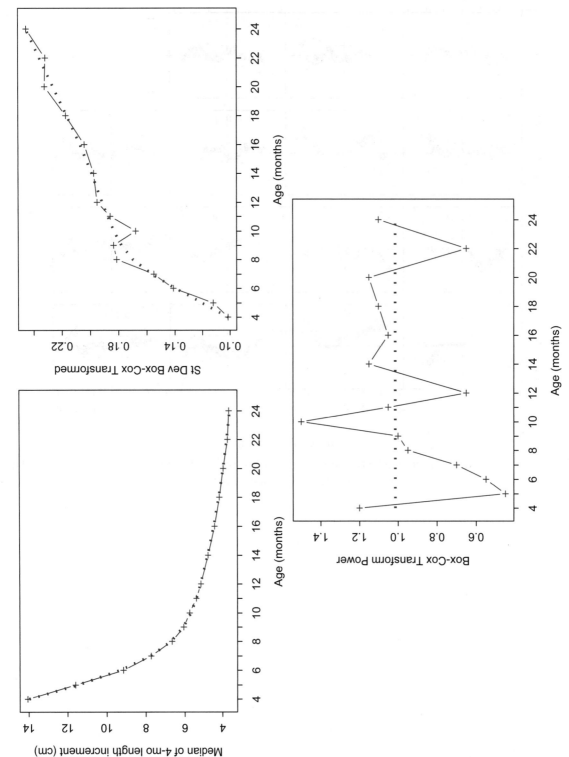

Figure A4.18 Fitting of the μ, σ, and ν curves of selected model for 4-month length velocity for boys

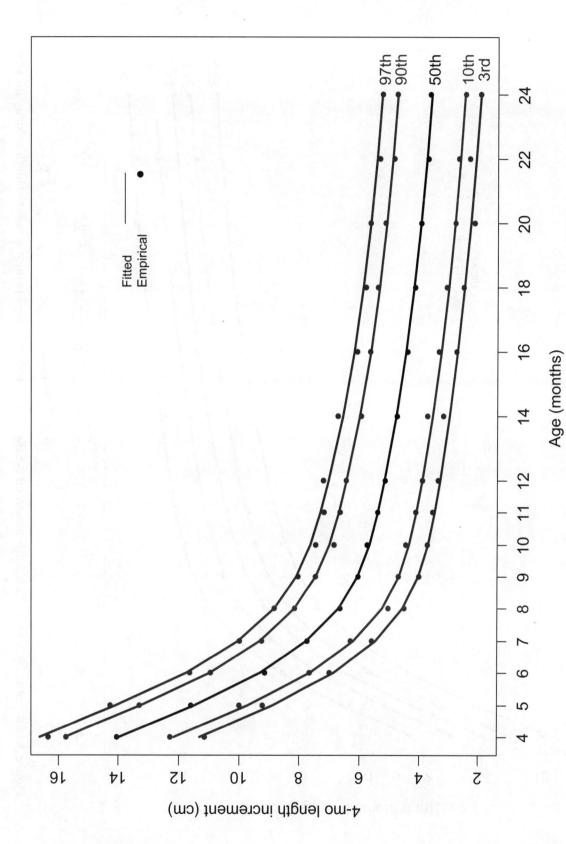

Figure A4.19 3rd, 10th, 50th, 90th, 97th smoothed centile curves and empirical values: 4-month length velocity for boys

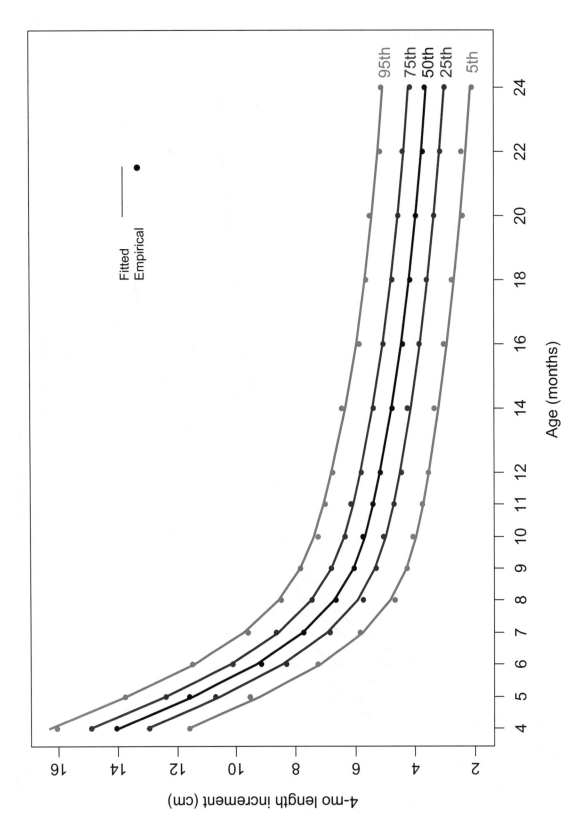

Figure A4.20 5th, 25th, 50th, 75th, 95th smoothed centile curves and empirical values: 4-month length velocity for boys

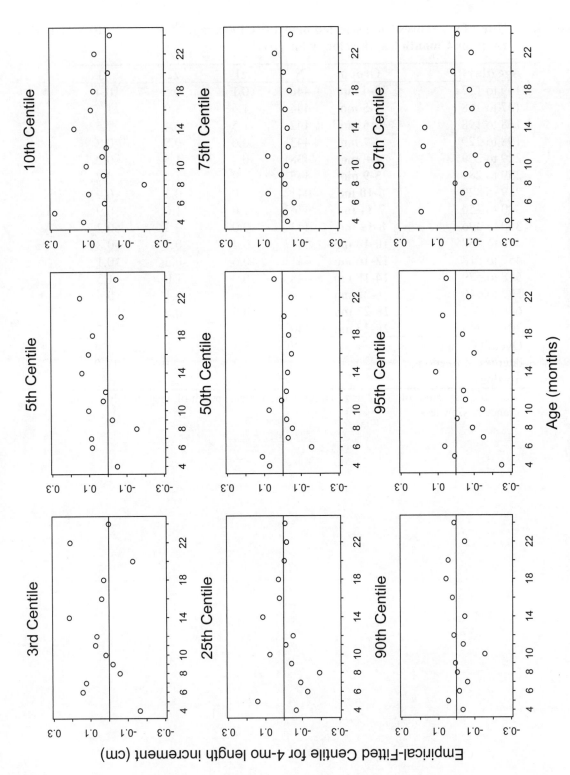

Figure A4.21 Centile residuals from fitting selected model for 4-month length velocity for boys

A4.3b 4-month intervals for girls

Table A4.4   **Q-test for z-scores from selected model [BCPE(x=age$^{0.05}$, df(μ)=8, df(σ)=5, df(v)=1, τ=2)] for 4-month length velocity for girls**

Age (days)	Group	N	z1	z2	z3
119 to 137	**0-4 mo**	446	0.1	0.5	0.4
137 to 168	**1-5 mo**	444	1.5	-1.0	1.7
168 to 198	**2-6 mo**	442	-1.5	-0.4	1.5
198 to 229	**3-7 mo**	443	0.6	-0.8	-0.8
229 to 259	**4-8 mo**	438	-0.7	1.5	-0.2
259 to 289	**5-9 mo**	445	-0.9	1.5	0.7
289 to 320	**6-10 mo**	441	0.0	-0.1	0.9
320 to 350	**7-11 mo**	436	1.0	-1.0	0.9
350 to 396	**8-12 mo**	443	0.0	-0.3	0.2
396 to 457	**10-14 mo**	444	0.4	-0.7	-0.8
457 to 518	**12-16 mo**	441	-0.6	-0.3	-0.1
518 to 579	**14-18 mo**	448	0.0	1.0	-1.3
579 to 640	**16-20 mo**	434	0.6	0.1	-0.5
640 to 701	**18-22 mo**	435	-0.5	0.0	-0.3
701 to 749	**20-24 mo**	440	0.0	-0.2	0.5
Overall Q stats		6620	8.5	9.2	11.4
degrees of freedom			7.0	12.0	14.0
p-value			0.2918	0.6849	0.6557

Note: Absolute values of z1, z2 or z3 larger than 2 indicate misfit of, respectively, mean, variance or skewness.

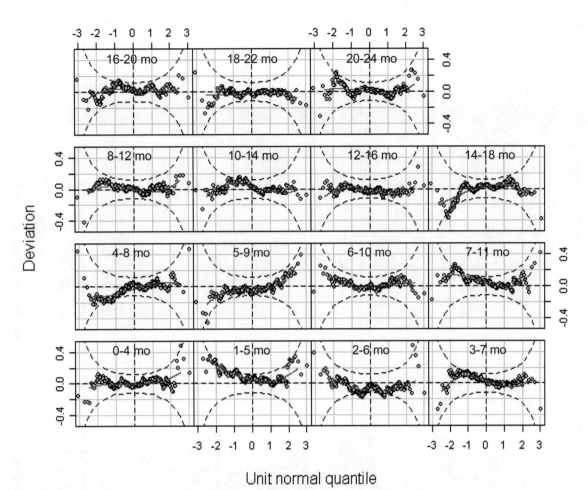

Figure A4.22 Worm plots from selected model [BCPE(x=age$^{0.05}$, df(μ)=8, df(σ)=5, df(ν)=1, τ=2)] for 4-month length velocity for girls

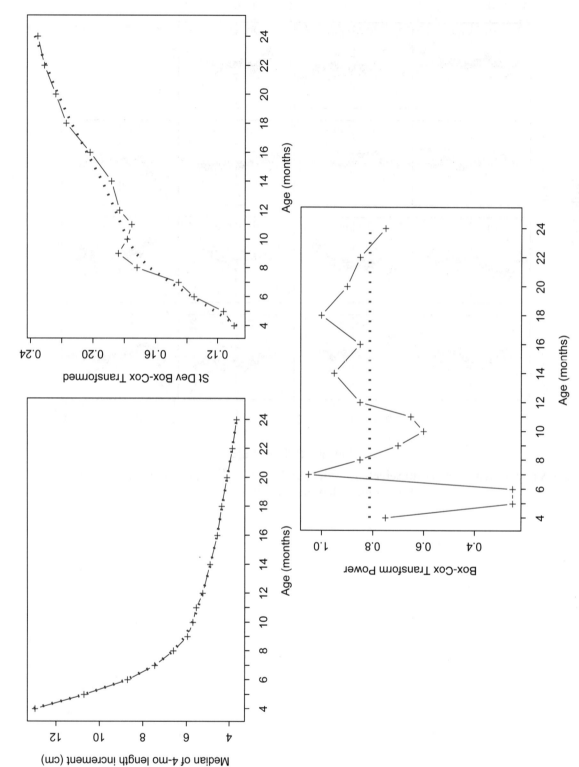

Figure A4.23 Fitting of the μ, σ, and ν curves of selected model for 4-month length velocity for girls

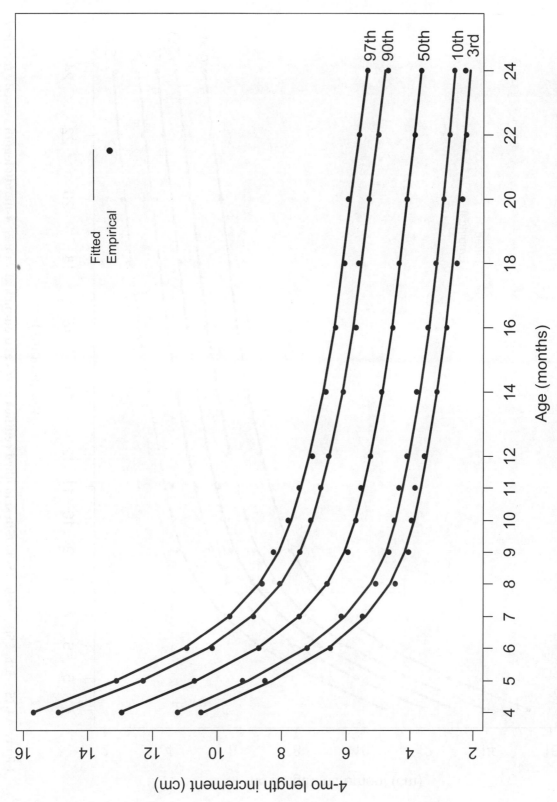

Figure A4.24   3rd, 10th, 50th, 90th, 97th smoothed centile curves and empirical values: 4-month length velocity for girls

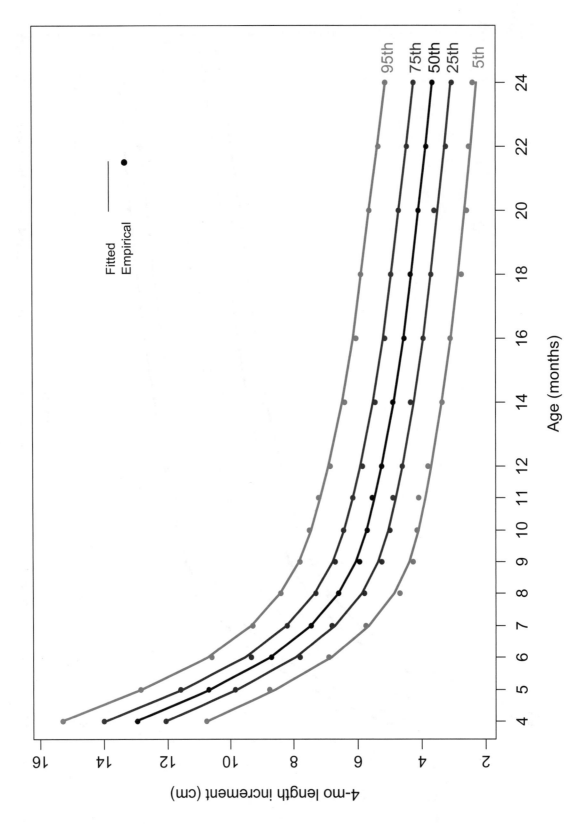

Figure A4.25   5th, 25th, 50th, 75th, 95th smoothed centile curves and empirical values: 4-month length velocity for girls

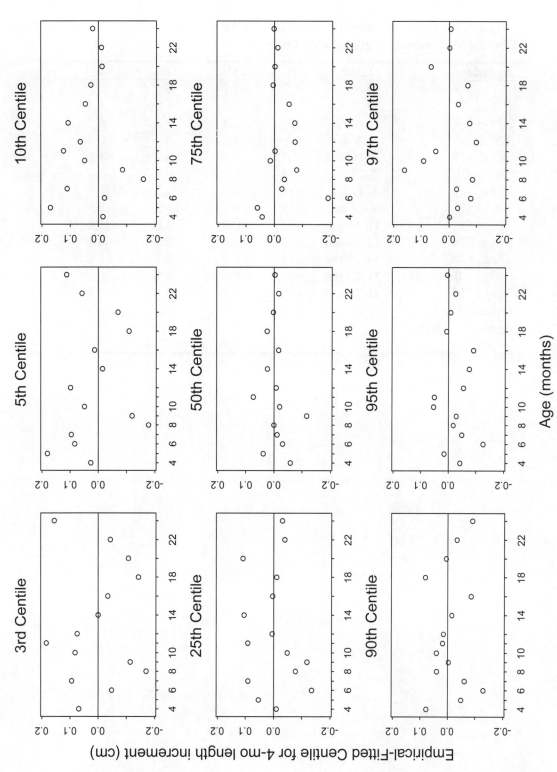

Figure A4.26 Centile residuals from fitting selected model for 4-month length velocity for girls

A4.4a 6-month intervals for boys

Table A4.5   Q-test for z-scores from selected model [BCPE(x=age$^{0.05}$, df(µ)=7, df(σ)=5, df(ν)=1, τ=2)] for 6-month length velocity for boys

Age (days)	Group	N	z1	z2	z3
175 to 198	**0-6 mo**	423	0.7	0.1	0.6
198 to 229	**1-7 mo**	417	1.5	-1.0	1.3
229 to 259	**2-8 mo**	416	-1.8	0.5	0.2
259 to 289	**3-9 mo**	409	-0.3	0.3	0.0
289 to 320	**4-10 mo**	403	-0.6	0.0	-1.2
320 to 350	**5-11 mo**	414	-0.1	0.7	-2.4
350 to 396	**6-12 mo**	419	-0.1	0.2	-1.5
396 to 457	**8-14 mo**	411	0.8	-0.5	-0.6
457 to 518	**10-16 mo**	402	0.0	-0.5	1.4
518 to 579	**12-18 mo**	411	0.4	-0.5	-0.1
579 to 640	**14-20 mo**	413	-0.8	1.2	1.7
640 to 701	**16-22 mo**	409	0.6	-1.1	0.1
701 to 750	**18-24 mo**	410	-0.3	0.5	1.6
Overall Q stats		5357	8.6	5.5	18.9
degrees of freedom			6.0	10.0	12.0
p-value			0.1963	0.8584	0.0920

Note: Absolute values of z1, z2 or z3 larger than 2 indicate misfit of, respectively, mean, variance or skewness.

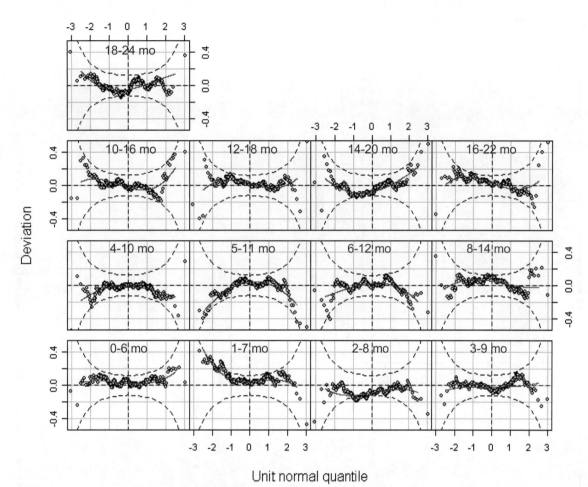

Unit normal quantile

Figure A4.27 Worm plots from selected model [BCPE(x=age$^{0.05}$, df(μ)=7, df(σ)=5, df(ν)=1, τ=2)] for 6-month length velocity for boys

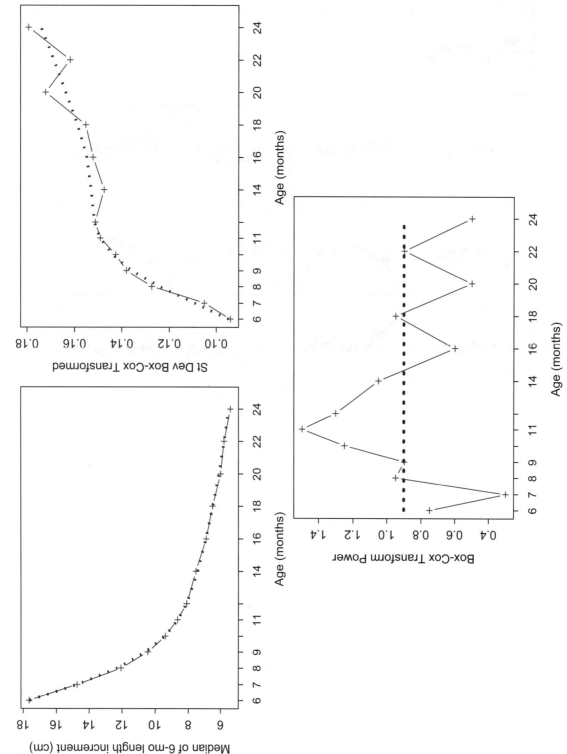

Figure A4. 28 Fitting of the μ, σ, and ν curves of selected model for 6-month length velocity for boys

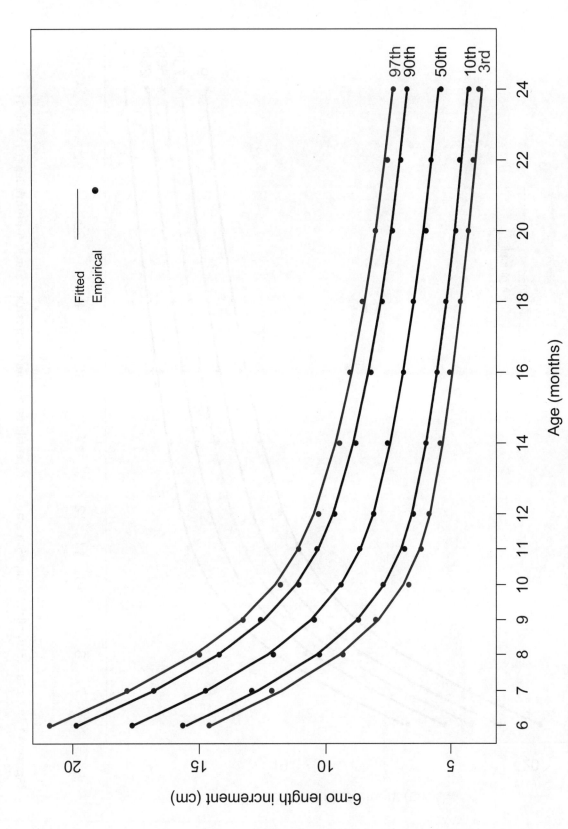

Figure A4.29   3rd, 10th, 50th, 90th, 97th smoothed centile curves and empirical values: 6-month length velocity for boys

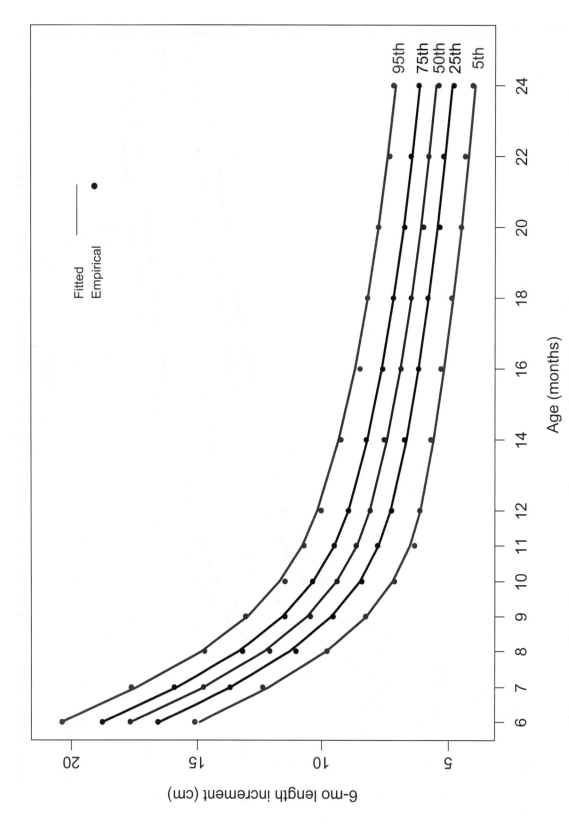

Figure A4.30   5th, 25th, 50th, 75th, 95th smoothed centile curves and empirical values: 6-month length velocity for boys

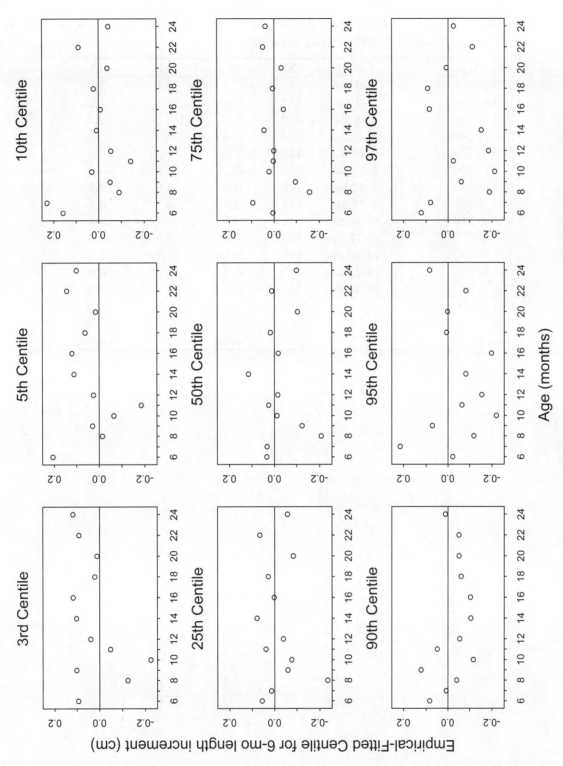

Figure A4.31 Centile residuals from fitting selected model for 6-month length velocity for boys

A4.4b 6-month intervals for girls

Table A4.6   Q-test for z-scores from selected model [BCPE(x=age$^{0.05}$, df(μ)=7, df(σ)=4, df(ν)=1, τ=2)] for 6-month length velocity for girls

Age (days)	Group	N	z1	z2	z3
178 to 198	**0-6 mo**	447	1.2	0.1	1.4
198 to 229	**1-7 mo**	442	0.6	-1.1	1.2
229 to 259	**2-8 mo**	439	-1.7	-0.1	0.7
259 to 289	**3-9 mo**	444	0.4	0.7	-0.6
289 to 320	**4-10 mo**	440	-1.1	1.2	0.8
320 to 350	**5-11 mo**	438	-0.3	0.4	-0.3
350 to 396	**6-12 mo**	446	0.6	-0.5	-0.1
396 to 457	**8-14 mo**	443	0.6	-0.3	0.5
457 to 518	**10-16 mo**	436	-0.1	-1.5	0.4
518 to 579	**12-18 mo**	447	-0.1	0.0	-1.0
579 to 640	**14-20 mo**	441	-0.1	1.7	-1.9
640 to 701	**16-22 mo**	430	0.4	-0.5	0.0
701 to 749	**18-24 mo**	446	-0.3	-0.2	1.3
Overall Q stats		5739	7.2	9.0	11.8
degrees of freedom			6.0	10.5	12.0
p-value			0.3058	0.5757	0.4646

Note: Absolute values of z1, z2 or z3 larger than 2 indicate misfit of, respectively, mean, variance or skewness.

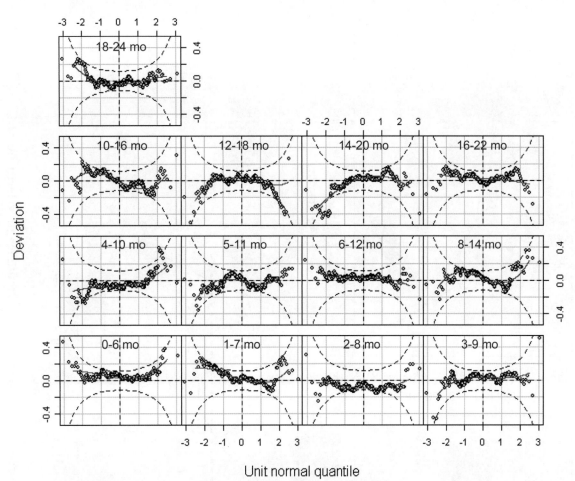

Unit normal quantile

Figure A4.32 Worm plots from selected model [BCPE(x=age$^{0.05}$, df(μ)=7, df(σ)=4, df(ν)=1, τ=2)] for 6-month length velocity for girls

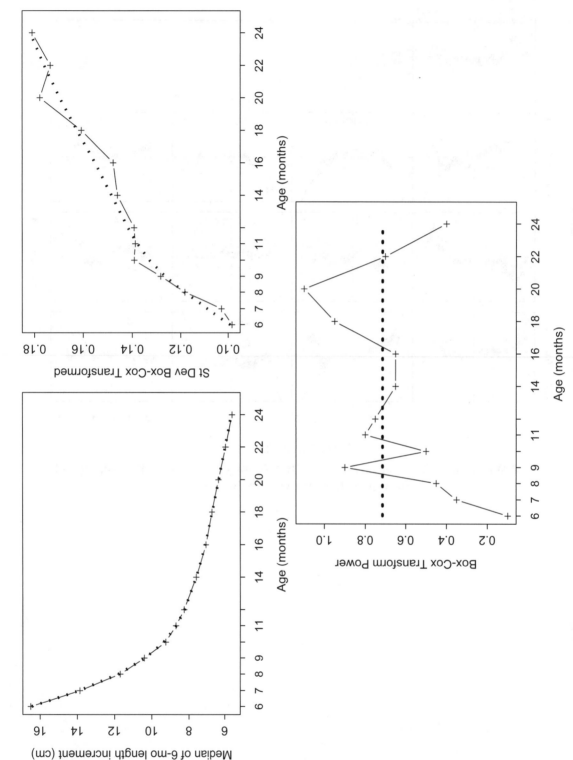

Figure A4.33 Fitting of the μ, σ, and ν curves of selected model for 6-month length velocity for girls

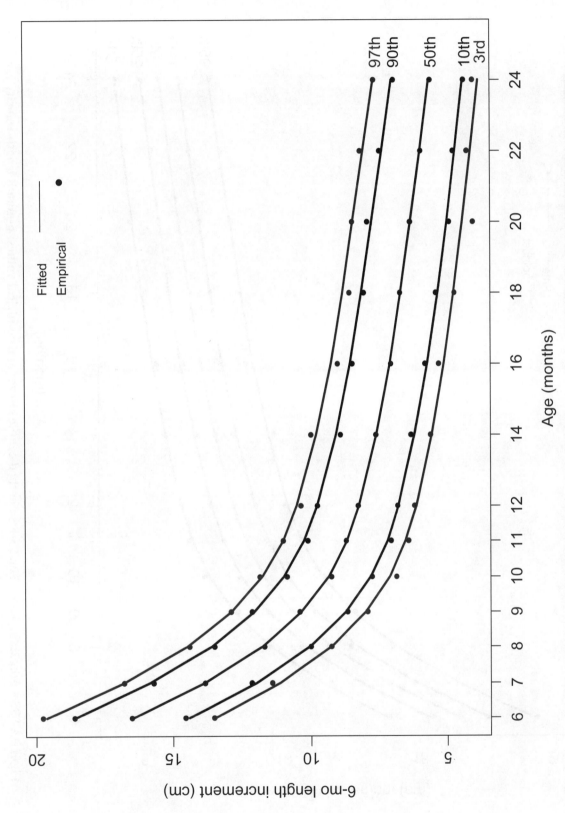

Figure A4.34 3rd, 10th, 50th, 90th, 97th smoothed centile curves and empirical values: 6-month length velocity for girls

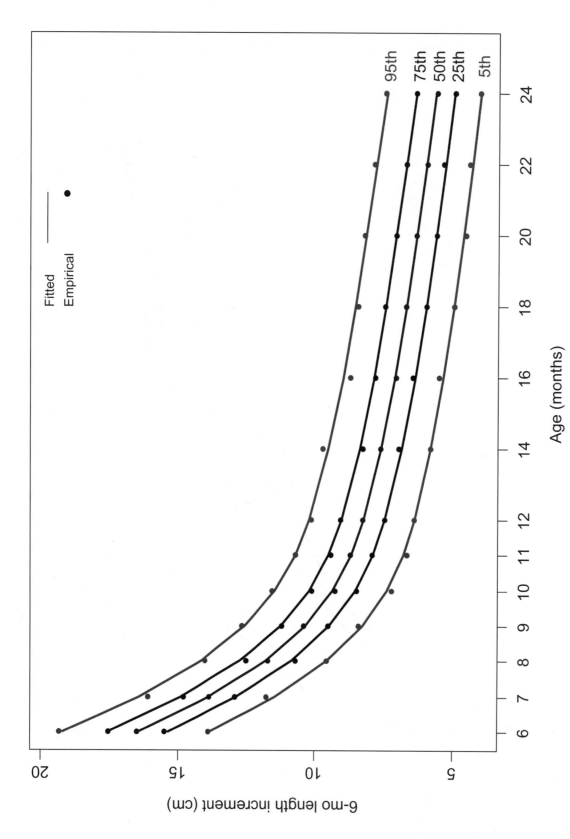

Figure A4.35   5th, 25th, 50th, 75th, 95th smoothed centile curves and empirical values: 6-month length velocity for girls

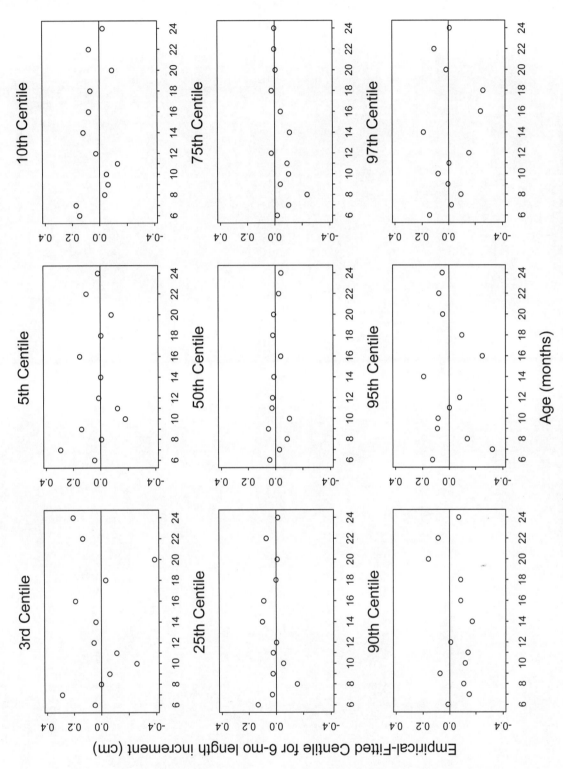

Figure A4.36 Centile residuals from fitting selected model for 6-month length velocity for girls

5. CONSTRUCTION OF THE HEAD CIRCUMFERENCE VELOCITY STANDARDS

The objective was to create sex-specific velocity curves for 2-, 3-, 4- and 6-month head circumference increments conditional on age. Tables generated from the 2-month increment curves provide estimated centiles for ages 0-2, 1-3, ..., 10-12 months; tables generated from the 3-month increment curves provide estimated centiles for ages 0-3, 1-4, ..., 9-12 months; tables generated from the 4-month increment curves provide estimated centiles for ages 0-4, 1-5, ..., 20-24 months; and tables generated from the 6-month increment curves provide estimated centiles for ages 0-6, 1-7, ..., 18-24 months. To avoid the right-edge effect, the 2- and 3-month intervals were modelled using data up to age 14 months.

By the same rationale applied to length increments, negative increments were recoded as "no growth" by assigning the nominal value of +0.01 to permit their inclusion in BCPE modelling. The numbers involved were: for the 2-month increments for boys 15 out of 4947 (0.30%) between -0.85 and -0.05 cm, and for girls 26 out of 5316 (0.49%) between -0.70 and -0.02 cm; for the 3-month increments for boys 4 out of 4536 (0.09%) between -0.30 and -0.05 cm and for girls 5 out of 4869 (0.10%) between -0.55 and -0.001 cm; for the 4-month increments for boys 19 out of 6178 (0.31%) between -0.30 and -0.008 cm, and for girls 24 out of 6629 (0.36%) between -0.45 and -0.05 cm; for the 6-month increments for boys 2 out of 5353 (0.04%) between -0.15 and -0.04 cm, and for girls 6 out of 5747 (0.10%) between -0.30 and -0.05 cm. As was the case for length, the effect of recoding the negative values on the final centiles was assessed using the girls' 2-month head circumference increments (the group with the largest number of negative increments). Comparisons between the model using the negative values (adding a delta value to all observations) and the model using recoded values showed that the recoding had no impact on the model specifications and results were comparable to those of length.

5.1   2-month intervals

Boys

There were 4947 2-month boys' head circumference increments from birth to 14 months. The best value of the age-transformation power was $\lambda=0.05$. The search for the best df(μ) and df(σ) followed, fixing $\lambda=0.05$, $\nu=1$ and $\tau=2$. Neither criterion GAIC(3) nor GAIC(4) was able to select the best degrees of freedom for the parameter μ. It was only with GAIC(5) that the search results indicated minima values. The model yielding the first smallest GAIC(5) was selected in favour of a smoother median curve. Thus, df(μ)=8 and df(σ)=4 were used to continue with a search for the best degrees of freedom to fit the parameter ν for skewness fixing $\tau=2$. The smallest GAIC(5) value corresponded to df(ν)=1 yet the ν curve using this was an under-smoothed fit of the empirical Box-Cox power values. Thus a choice was made to use df(ν)=4, which was primarily supported by criteria GAIC(3) and GAIC(4), and the model BCPE(x=age$^{0.05}$, df(μ)=8, df(σ)=4, df(ν)=4, τ=2) was further evaluated.

The diagnostic results are presented in Appendix A5, section A5.1a. The overall Q-test p-values (Table A5.1) indicate an adequate fit of the parameters μ and σ (p-values > 0.05) with residual skewness (absolute z3 values > 2) in only one out of 12 age groups (7-9 mo). The worm plots (Figure A5.1) from this model agree with the Q-test results. The fitted curves of the parameters μ, σ and ν seemed adequate when compared to the empirical values (Figure A5.2). The fitted centile curves and empirical centiles are shown in figures A5.3 and A5.4, and they indicate close concordance between the two. Figure A5.5 shows the distribution of empirical minus fitted centile differences with no evidence of systematic bias except for a slight over-estimation of the 75th, 90th and 95th centiles by about 0.05 cm.

Table 26 presents the predicted centiles for boys' 2-month head circumference velocities between birth and 12 months.

Girls

There were 5316 girls' 2-month head circumference increments from birth to 14 months. The best value of the age-transformation power was $\lambda=0.05$. The search for the best df(μ) and df(σ) followed, fixing $\lambda=0.05$, $v=1$ and $\tau=2$. The GAIC(3) reached more than one local minima, the first occurring for the model with df(μ)=8 and df(σ)=4. The next minimum for the GAIC(3) was yielded by a model of considerably higher degrees of freedom and lesser smoothness (df(μ)=11 and df(σ)=4). In favour of greater smoothness, the model with df(μ)=8 and df(σ)=4 was further examined and the next step was to search for the best degrees of freedom to fit the parameter v for skewness fixing $\tau=2$. The smallest GAIC(3) value corresponded to df(v)=1 and the model BCPE($x=age^{0.05}$, df(μ)=8, df(σ)=4, df(v)=1, $\tau=2$) was further evaluated.

The diagnostic test results are presented in Appendix A5, section A5.1b. For the selected model, the Q-test results (Table A5.2) show overall Q-test for μ and σ with p-values above 0.05 indicating an adequate fit of these parameters. For the parameter v, the overall Q-test was significant indicating residual skewness (absolute z3 values > 2) in two out of 12 age groups. The worm plots (Figure A5.6) show similar results to those of the Q-test. Figure A5.7 displays the fitted curves of the parameters μ and σ, which closely followed the respective empirical point estimates; the model fitting a constant for the parameter v also approximates fairly well the fluctuations observed empirically. Similar to the boys, comparisons between fitted and empirical centiles are in close agreement, and centile residuals depict slight over-estimation by about 0.05 cm of the 75th and higher centiles (Figures A5.8 to A5.10).

Table 27 presents the predicted centiles for girls' 2-month head circumference velocities between birth and 12 months.

5.2   3-month intervals

Boys

There were 4536 boys' 3-month observed head circumference increments from birth to 14 months. The best value of the age-transformation power was $\lambda=0.05$. The search for the best df(μ) and df(σ) followed, fixing $\lambda=0.05$, $v=1$ and $\tau=2$. Once more, the GAIC(3) reached more than one local minima values, the first occurring for the model with df(μ)=7 and df(σ)=4. The next minimum for the GAIC(3) came from a model of considerably higher degrees of freedom and lesser smoothness (df(μ)=13 and df(σ)=4). To maintain the smoother fit (with the lower degrees of freedom for μ), the model with df(μ)=7 and df(σ)=4 was selected, followed by the search for the best degrees of freedom to fit the parameter v for skewness fixing $\tau=2$. The smallest GAIC(3) value corresponded to df(v)=4 and the model BCPE($x=age^{0.05}$, df(μ)=7, df(σ)=4, df(v)=4 , $\tau=2$) was further evaluated.

The diagnostic results are presented in Appendix A5, section A5.2a. In Table A5.3, the overall Q-test p-values for the median, variance and skewness were all non-significant, indicating an adequate fit of the boys' 3-month head circumference increments. Similarly, the worm plots shown in Figure A5.11 of the selected model indicate an adequate fit of the data. There was no evident bias when comparing fitted μ, σ and v parameter curves with their respective sample estimates (Figure A5.12). Figures A5.13 to A5.15 show no sizeable bias comparing the empirical and fitted centiles, and the centile residuals.

Table 28 presents the predicted centiles for boys' 3-month head circumference velocities between birth and 12 months.

Girls

There were 4869 girls' 3-month observed head circumference increments from birth to 14 months. The best value of the age-transformation power was $\lambda=0.05$. The search for the best $df(\mu)$ and $df(\sigma)$ followed, fixing $\lambda=0.05$, $\nu=1$ and $\tau=2$. Using GAIC(3) there was no minimum value and that was also the case when the penalty was raised to 4. With penalty 5 (GAIC(5)) the first occurring minimum value was associated with the model with $df(\mu)=7$ and $df(\sigma)=4$. Next, the GAIC(5) indicated a smaller value only with considerably higher degrees of freedom and lesser smoothness ($df(\mu)=15$ or higher and $df(\sigma)=4$). Thus, the model with $df(\mu)=7$ and $df(\sigma)=4$ was used to search for the best degrees of freedom to fit the parameter ν for skewness fixing $\tau=2$. The smallest GAIC(3) value corresponded to $df(\nu)=4$, while the smallest GAIC(5) indicated $df(\nu)=2$. The choice that provided the smoother ν curve, i.e. $df(\nu)=2$, was selected and the model BCPE($x=age^{0.05}$, $df(\mu)=7$, $df(\sigma)=4$, $df(\nu)=2$, $\tau=2$) was further evaluated.

The diagnostic test results are presented in Appendix A5, section A5.2b. In Table A5.4, the overall Q-test for the median parameter μ was significant, but none of the z1 values exceed absolute value 2, and the same applied to the skewness parameter ν (2 out of 11 z3 values exceed absolute value 2). The overall significance, especially for the median might be due in part to the small number of age groups (11) for this interval relative to the number of degrees of freedom necessary for fitting the parameter, which leaves a small number of degrees of freedom for the overall Q-test statistics. The worm plots (Figure A5.16) confirm findings of the Q-tests (i.e. one group with a U-shaped worm and another with an inverted U-shaped worm). Examining figure A5.17 of the fitted parameters, there were fluctuations notably in the empirical curve of the parameter ν that were smoothed out by the selected model. The adequacy of the fitted model was indicated by the comparisons between fitted and empirical centiles (A5.18 and A5.19) and centile residuals (A5.20), the latter showing an average under-estimation of 0.05 cm in the 10th centile and an equally negligible over-estimation in the 90th centile.

Table 29 presents the predicted centiles for girls' 3-month head circumference velocities between birth and 12 months.

5.3   4-month intervals

Boys

There were 6178 boys' 4-month head circumference increments from birth to 24 months, one of which was excluded as an outlier, leaving a final sample of 6177 observations for the modeling exercise. The best value of the age-transformation power was $\lambda=0.05$. The search for the best $df(\mu)$ and $df(\sigma)$ followed, fixing $\lambda=0.05$, $\nu=1$ and $\tau=2$. The model with $df(\mu)=10$ and $df(\sigma)=5$ provided the smallest GAIC(3). The next step was to search for the best degrees of freedom to fit the parameter ν for skewness fixing $\tau=2$ and keeping the degrees of freedom for the previously selected μ and σ curves. The smallest GAIC(3) value corresponded to $df(\nu)=3$. Hence, the model BCPE($x=age^{0.05}$, $df(\mu)=10$, $df(\sigma)=5$, $df(\nu)=3$, $\tau=2$) was selected and further evaluated.

The diagnostic test results are presented in Appendix A5, section A5.3a. The Q-test results (Table A5.5) and worm plots (Figure A5.21) from this model indicated an adequate fit of the data with the overall Q-test p-values for the three parameters being non-significant at the 5% level. Figure A5.22 shows the fitted μ, σ and ν curves against their corresponding empirical estimates. Notably, the ν parameter empirical curve exhibits fluctuations which are reasonably smoothed by the fitted curve. The next three plots (figures A5.23, A5.24 and A5.25) show no evidence of bias when comparing fitted against empirical centiles or centile residuals, except for a slight over-estimation in the 75th, 90th and 95th centiles by about 0.05 cm.

Table 30 presents the predicted centiles for boys' 4-month head circumference velocities between birth and 24 months.

Girls

There were 6629 girls' 4-month head circumference increments from birth to 24 months, one of which was excluded as an outlier, leaving a final sample of 6628 observations for the modeling exercise. The best value of the age-transformation power was $\lambda=0.05$. The search for the best df(μ) and df(σ) followed, fixing $\lambda=0.05$, $\nu=1$ and $\tau=2$. The model with df(μ)=10 and df(σ)=5 provided the smallest GAIC(3). The next step was to search for the best degrees of freedom to fit the parameter ν for skewness fixing $\tau=2$ and keeping the degrees of freedom for the previously selected μ and σ curves. The smallest GAIC(3) value corresponded to df(ν)=2 and the model BCPE(x=age$^{0.05}$, df(μ)=10, df(σ)=5, df(ν)=2, $\tau=2$) was further evaluated.

The diagnostic test results are presented in Appendix A5, section A5.3b. The overall Q-test p-values (in Table A5.6) indicate an adequate fit of the median parameter μ and σ curves. For the skewness parameter ν although the overall Q-test was significant, residual skewness occurred in only two out of 15 age groups. The worm plots (Figure A5.26) from this model reflect residual skewness in the same age group as indicated by the Q-test results. Figure A5.27 shows adequate fitting of the parameters μ and σ with the respective sample estimates and a reasonable smoothing of the fluctuations in the empirical curve for ν by the selected model. Comparisons between fitted and empirical centiles and centile residuals depict a reasonable fit of the data (Figures A5.28 and A5.29) with a slight under-estimation in the 10th centile by about 0.05 cm and a similar over-estimation in the 75th and higher centiles (Figure A5.30).

Table 31 presents the predicted centiles for girls' 4-month head circumference velocities between birth and 24 months.

5.4   6-month intervals

Boys

There were 5353 boys' 6-month head circumference increments from birth to 24 months, one of which was excluded as an outlier, leaving a final sample of 5352 observations for the modelling exercise. The best value of the age-transformation power was $\lambda=0.05$. The search for the best df(μ) and df(σ) followed, fixing $\lambda=0.05$, $\nu=1$ and $\tau=2$. The model with df(μ)=9 and df(σ)=4 provided the smallest GAIC(3). The next step was to search for the best degrees of freedom to fit the parameter ν for skewness fixing $\tau=2$ and keeping the degrees of freedom for the previously selected μ and σ curves. The smallest GAIC(3) value corresponded to df(ν)=2. Hence, the model BCPE(x=age$^{0.05}$, df(μ)=9, df(σ)=4, df(ν)=2, $\tau=2$) was selected and further evaluated.

The diagnostic test results are presented in Appendix A5, section A5.4a. The Q-test results (Table A5.7) and worm plots (Figure A5.31) from this model indicated an adequate fit of the data with the overall Q-test p-values for the three parameters being non-significant at the 5% level. Figure A5.32 shows the fitted μ, σ and ν curves against their corresponding empirical estimates. The ν parameter fitted curve smoothes out reasonably well the fluctuations exhibited by the empirical curve. Figures A5.33, A5.34 and A5.35 show some evidence of bias in the comparison of fitted against empirical centiles and centile residual plots at the lowest centiles (between the 3rd and the 10th centiles) but the magnitude of the biases is negligible.

Table 32 presents the predicted centiles for boys' 6-month head circumference velocities between birth and 24 months.

Girls

There were 5747 girls' 6-month head circumference increments from birth to 24 months, one of which was excluded as an outlier, leaving a final sample of 5746 observations for the modelling exercise. The best value of the age-transformation power was λ=0.05. The search for the best df(μ) and df(σ) followed, fixing λ=0.05, ν=1 and τ=2. The model with df(μ)=9 and df(σ)=5 provided the smallest GAIC(3). The next step was to search for the best degrees of freedom to fit the parameter ν for skewness fixing τ=2 and keeping the degrees of freedom for the previously selected μ and σ curves. The smallest GAIC(3) value corresponded to df(ν)=2 and the model BCPE(x=age$^{0.05}$, df(μ)=9, df(σ)=5, df(ν)=2, τ=2) was further evaluated.

The diagnostic test results are presented in Appendix A5, section A5.4b. Table A5.8 summarizes Q-test results, indicating an adequate fit of the median and skewness parameters and a slight misfit of the σ parameter curve in the last two age groups (out of 13). The overall Q-test p-values were all non-significant. The worm plots (Figure A5.36) from this model partially reflect the variance misfit in one age group (18-24 mo). Figure A5.37 shows adequate fitting of the three parameters μ, σ and ν by the selected model. Comparisons between fitted and empirical centiles and the centile residuals depict a reasonable fit of the data (Figures A5.38 to A5.40). Similar to boys, there is a slight indication of bias but the magnitude also is negligible.

Table 33 presents the predicted centiles for girls' 6-month head circumference velocities between birth and 24 months.

Table 26 Boys 2-month head circumference increments (cm)

Interval	L	M	S	1st	3rd	5th	15th	25th	50th	75th	85th	95th	97th	99th
0-2 mo	0.9267	4.6878	0.16093	3.0	3.3	3.5	3.9	4.2	4.7	5.2	5.5	5.9	6.1	6.5
1-3 mo	0.6210	3.3714	0.15634	2.2	2.4	2.5	2.8	3.0	3.4	3.7	3.9	4.3	4.4	4.7
2-4 mo	0.5607	2.5170	0.16382	1.6	1.8	1.9	2.1	2.2	2.5	2.8	3.0	3.2	3.3	3.6
3-5 mo	0.6219	2.0747	0.18097	1.3	1.4	1.5	1.7	1.8	2.1	2.3	2.5	2.7	2.8	3.0
4-6 mo	0.7141	1.7184	0.20700	1.0	1.1	1.2	1.4	1.5	1.7	2.0	2.1	2.3	2.4	2.6
5-7 mo	0.7879	1.4381	0.23798	0.7	0.8	0.9	1.1	1.2	1.4	1.7	1.8	2.0	2.1	2.3
6-8 mo	0.8482	1.2009	0.27392	0.5	0.6	0.7	0.9	1.0	1.2	1.4	1.5	1.8	1.8	2.0
7-9 mo	0.8985	1.0106	0.31173	0.3	0.4	0.5	0.7	0.8	1.0	1.2	1.3	1.5	1.6	1.8
8-10 mo	0.9379	0.8731	0.35212	0.2	0.3	0.4	0.6	0.7	0.9	1.1	1.2	1.4	1.5	1.6
9-11 mo	0.9577	0.7615	0.39591	0.1	0.2	0.3	0.5	0.6	0.8	1.0	1.1	1.3	1.3	1.5
10-12 mo	0.9598	0.6659	0.44007	0.0	0.1	0.2	0.4	0.5	0.7	0.9	1.0	1.2	1.2	1.4

Interval	L	M	S	-3SD	-2SD	-1SD	Median	+1SD	+2SD	+3SD
0-2 mo	0.9267	4.6878	0.16093	2.5	3.2	3.9	4.7	5.4	6.2	7.0
1-3 mo	0.6210	3.3714	0.15634	1.9	2.4	2.9	3.4	3.9	4.5	5.1
2-4 mo	0.5607	2.5170	0.16382	1.4	1.8	2.1	2.5	2.9	3.4	3.9
3-5 mo	0.6219	2.0747	0.18097	1.1	1.4	1.7	2.1	2.5	2.9	3.3
4-6 mo	0.7141	1.7184	0.20700	0.8	1.1	1.4	1.7	2.1	2.5	2.9
5-7 mo	0.7879	1.4381	0.23798	0.5	0.8	1.1	1.4	1.8	2.2	2.5
6-8 mo	0.8482	1.2009	0.27392	0.3	0.6	0.9	1.2	1.5	1.9	2.2
7-9 mo	0.8985	1.0106	0.31173	0.1	0.4	0.7	1.0	1.3	1.7	2.0
8-10 mo	0.9379	0.8731	0.35212	0.0	0.3	0.6	0.9	1.2	1.5	1.8
9-11 mo	0.9577	0.7615	0.39591	0.0	0.2	0.5	0.8	1.1	1.4	1.7
10-12 mo	0.9598	0.6659	0.44007	0.0	0.1	0.4	0.7	1.0	1.3	1.6

Table 27 Girls 2-month head circumference increments (cm)

Interval	L	M	S	1st	3rd	5th	15th	25th	50th	75th	85th	95th	97th	99th
0-2 mo	0.8807	4.3539	0.15953	2.8	3.1	3.2	3.6	3.9	4.4	4.8	5.1	5.5	5.7	6.0
1-3 mo	0.8807	3.1035	0.16706	1.9	2.1	2.3	2.6	2.8	3.1	3.5	3.6	4.0	4.1	4.3
2-4 mo	0.8807	2.3473	0.18107	1.4	1.6	1.7	1.9	2.1	2.3	2.6	2.8	3.1	3.2	3.4
3-5 mo	0.8807	1.9599	0.20017	1.1	1.2	1.3	1.6	1.7	2.0	2.2	2.4	2.6	2.7	2.9
4-6 mo	0.8807	1.6524	0.22476	0.8	1.0	1.1	1.3	1.4	1.7	1.9	2.0	2.3	2.4	2.5
5-7 mo	0.8807	1.3981	0.25281	0.6	0.8	0.8	1.0	1.2	1.4	1.6	1.8	2.0	2.1	2.2
6-8 mo	0.8807	1.1762	0.28607	0.4	0.6	0.6	0.8	1.0	1.2	1.4	1.5	1.7	1.8	2.0
7-9 mo	0.8807	0.9921	0.32161	0.3	0.4	0.5	0.7	0.8	1.0	1.2	1.3	1.5	1.6	1.8
8-10 mo	0.8807	0.8471	0.35933	0.2	0.3	0.4	0.5	0.6	0.8	1.1	1.2	1.4	1.4	1.6
9-11 mo	0.8807	0.7384	0.40034	0.1	0.2	0.3	0.4	0.5	0.7	0.9	1.1	1.2	1.3	1.5
10-12 mo	0.8807	0.6552	0.44193	0.0	0.1	0.2	0.4	0.5	0.7	0.9	1.0	1.1	1.2	1.4

Interval	L	M	S	-3SD	-2SD	-1SD	Median	+1SD	+2SD	+3SD
0-2 mo	0.8807	4.3539	0.15953	2.3	3.0	3.7	4.4	5.1	5.8	6.5
1-3 mo	0.8807	3.1035	0.16706	1.6	2.1	2.6	3.1	3.6	4.2	4.7
2-4 mo	0.8807	2.3473	0.18107	1.1	1.5	1.9	2.3	2.8	3.2	3.7
3-5 mo	0.8807	1.9599	0.20017	0.8	1.2	1.6	2.0	2.4	2.8	3.2
4-6 mo	0.8807	1.6524	0.22476	0.6	0.9	1.3	1.7	2.0	2.4	2.8
5-7 mo	0.8807	1.3981	0.25281	0.4	0.7	1.1	1.4	1.8	2.1	2.5
6-8 mo	0.8807	1.1762	0.28607	0.2	0.5	0.8	1.2	1.5	1.9	2.2
7-9 mo	0.8807	0.9921	0.32161	0.1	0.4	0.7	1.0	1.3	1.7	2.0
8-10 mo	0.8807	0.8471	0.35933	0.0	0.3	0.5	0.8	1.2	1.5	1.8
9-11 mo	0.8807	0.7384	0.40034	0.0	0.2	0.5	0.7	1.0	1.4	1.7
10-12 mo	0.8807	0.6552	0.44193	0.0	0.1	0.4	0.7	1.0	1.3	1.6

Table 28　Boys 3-month head circumference increments (cm)

Interval	L	M	S	1st	3rd	5th	15th	25th	50th	75th	85th	95th	97th	99th
0-3 mo	0.7558	6.0419	0.13725	4.2	4.5	4.7	5.2	5.5	6.0	6.6	6.9	7.4	7.6	8.0
1-4 mo	0.4737	4.5132	0.13624	3.2	3.4	3.6	3.9	4.1	4.5	4.9	5.2	5.6	5.7	6.1
2-5 mo	0.4137	3.4944	0.14382	2.4	2.6	2.7	3.0	3.2	3.5	3.8	4.0	4.4	4.5	4.8
3-6 mo	0.4858	2.8568	0.15846	1.9	2.1	2.2	2.4	2.6	2.9	3.2	3.3	3.7	3.8	4.0
4-7 mo	0.5992	2.3840	0.17799	1.5	1.6	1.7	2.0	2.1	2.4	2.7	2.8	3.1	3.2	3.5
5-8 mo	0.7074	1.9903	0.20021	1.1	1.3	1.4	1.6	1.7	2.0	2.3	2.4	2.7	2.8	3.0
6-9 mo	0.8123	1.6704	0.22358	0.8	1.0	1.1	1.3	1.4	1.7	1.9	2.1	2.3	2.4	2.6
7-10 mo	0.9028	1.4214	0.24758	0.6	0.8	0.9	1.1	1.2	1.4	1.7	1.8	2.0	2.1	2.3
8-11 mo	0.9602	1.2321	0.27193	0.5	0.6	0.7	0.9	1.0	1.2	1.5	1.6	1.8	1.9	2.0
9-12 mo	0.9852	1.0768	0.29648	0.3	0.5	0.6	0.7	0.9	1.1	1.3	1.4	1.6	1.7	1.8

Interval	L	M	S	-3SD	-2SD	-1SD	Median	+1SD	+2SD	+3SD
0-3 mo	0.7558	6.0419	0.13725	3.7	4.4	5.2	6.0	6.9	7.8	8.6
1-4 mo	0.4737	4.5132	0.13624	2.9	3.4	3.9	4.5	5.2	5.8	6.6
2-5 mo	0.4137	3.4944	0.14382	2.2	2.6	3.0	3.5	4.0	4.6	5.2
3-6 mo	0.4858	2.8568	0.15846	1.7	2.0	2.4	2.9	3.3	3.8	4.4
4-7 mo	0.5992	2.3840	0.17799	1.3	1.6	2.0	2.4	2.8	3.3	3.8
5-8 mo	0.7074	1.9903	0.20021	0.9	1.2	1.6	2.0	2.4	2.8	3.3
6-9 mo	0.8123	1.6704	0.22358	0.6	1.0	1.3	1.7	2.1	2.4	2.9
7-10 mo	0.9028	1.4214	0.24758	0.4	0.7	1.1	1.4	1.8	2.1	2.5
8-11 mo	0.9602	1.2321	0.27193	0.3	0.6	0.9	1.2	1.6	1.9	2.3
9-12 mo	0.9852	1.0768	0.29648	0.1	0.4	0.8	1.1	1.4	1.7	2.0

Table 29 Girls 3-month head circumference increments (cm)

Interval	L	M	S	1st	3rd	5th	15th	25th	50th	75th	85th	95th	97th	99th
0-3 mo	0.4252	5.5822	0.14155	3.9	4.2	4.4	4.8	5.1	5.6	6.1	6.4	7.0	7.2	7.6
1-4 mo	0.5408	4.1837	0.14611	2.9	3.1	3.2	3.6	3.8	4.2	4.6	4.8	5.2	5.4	5.7
2-5 mo	0.6316	3.2594	0.15573	2.2	2.4	2.5	2.7	2.9	3.3	3.6	3.8	4.1	4.3	4.5
3-6 mo	0.7066	2.7161	0.16952	1.7	1.9	2.0	2.3	2.4	2.7	3.0	3.2	3.5	3.6	3.8
4-7 mo	0.7704	2.2991	0.18602	1.4	1.5	1.6	1.9	2.0	2.3	2.6	2.8	3.0	3.1	3.3
5-8 mo	0.8262	1.9451	0.20505	1.1	1.2	1.3	1.5	1.7	1.9	2.2	2.4	2.6	2.7	2.9
6-9 mo	0.8756	1.6363	0.22644	0.8	1.0	1.0	1.3	1.4	1.6	1.9	2.0	2.3	2.3	2.5
7-10 mo	0.9201	1.3903	0.24920	0.6	0.8	0.8	1.0	1.2	1.4	1.6	1.8	2.0	2.1	2.2
8-11 mo	0.9605	1.2025	0.27282	0.5	0.6	0.7	0.9	1.0	1.2	1.4	1.5	1.7	1.8	2.0
9-12 mo	0.9976	1.0690	0.29743	0.3	0.5	0.5	0.7	0.9	1.1	1.3	1.4	1.6	1.7	1.8

Interval	L	M	S	-3SD	-2SD	-1SD	Median	+1SD	+2SD	+3SD
0-3 mo	0.4252	5.5822	0.14155	3.5	4.1	4.8	5.6	6.4	7.3	8.2
1-4 mo	0.5408	4.1837	0.14611	2.5	3.0	3.6	4.2	4.8	5.5	6.2
2-5 mo	0.6316	3.2594	0.15573	1.9	2.3	2.8	3.3	3.8	4.3	4.9
3-6 mo	0.7066	2.7161	0.16952	1.4	1.8	2.3	2.7	3.2	3.7	4.2
4-7 mo	0.7704	2.2991	0.18602	1.1	1.5	1.9	2.3	2.7	3.2	3.7
5-8 mo	0.8262	1.9451	0.20505	0.8	1.2	1.6	1.9	2.4	2.8	3.2
6-9 mo	0.8756	1.6363	0.22644	0.6	0.9	1.3	1.6	2.0	2.4	2.8
7-10 mo	0.9201	1.3903	0.24920	0.4	0.7	1.0	1.4	1.7	2.1	2.5
8-11 mo	0.9605	1.2025	0.27282	0.2	0.6	0.9	1.2	1.5	1.9	2.2
9-12 mo	0.9976	1.0690	0.29743	0.1	0.4	0.8	1.1	1.4	1.7	2.0

Table 30 Boys 4-month head circumference increments (cm)

Interval	L	M	S	1st	3rd	5th	15th	25th	50th	75th	85th	95th	97th	99th
0-4 mo	0.3279	7.1133	0.12440	5.2	5.6	5.8	6.2	6.5	7.1	7.7	8.1	8.7	8.9	9.4
1-5 mo	0.4212	5.4806	0.12713	4.0	4.3	4.4	4.8	5.0	5.5	6.0	6.2	6.7	6.9	7.2
2-6 mo	0.5076	4.2702	0.13454	3.0	3.3	3.4	3.7	3.9	4.3	4.7	4.9	5.3	5.4	5.7
3-7 mo	0.5840	3.5185	0.14592	2.4	2.6	2.7	3.0	3.2	3.5	3.9	4.1	4.4	4.5	4.8
4-8 mo	0.6557	2.9255	0.16106	1.9	2.1	2.2	2.5	2.6	2.9	3.2	3.4	3.7	3.9	4.1
5-9 mo	0.7179	2.4506	0.17841	1.5	1.7	1.8	2.0	2.2	2.5	2.8	2.9	3.2	3.3	3.5
6-10 mo	0.7719	2.0780	0.19784	1.2	1.3	1.4	1.7	1.8	2.1	2.4	2.5	2.8	2.9	3.1
7-11 mo	0.8180	1.7696	0.21918	0.9	1.1	1.2	1.4	1.5	1.8	2.0	2.2	2.4	2.5	2.7
8-12 mo	0.8532	1.5301	0.24082	0.7	0.9	0.9	1.2	1.3	1.5	1.8	1.9	2.2	2.2	2.4
9-13 mo	0.8808	1.3368	0.26394	0.6	0.7	0.8	1.0	1.1	1.3	1.6	1.7	1.9	2.0	2.2
10-14 mo	0.9009	1.1844	0.28656	0.4	0.6	0.6	0.8	1.0	1.2	1.4	1.5	1.8	1.8	2.0
11-15 mo	0.9166	1.0457	0.30970	0.3	0.5	0.5	0.7	0.8	1.0	1.3	1.4	1.6	1.7	1.8
12-16 mo	0.9278	0.9301	0.33162	0.2	0.4	0.4	0.6	0.7	0.9	1.1	1.3	1.4	1.5	1.7
13-17 mo	0.9357	0.8359	0.35292	0.2	0.3	0.4	0.5	0.6	0.8	1.0	1.1	1.3	1.4	1.5
14-18 mo	0.9414	0.7605	0.37421	0.1	0.2	0.3	0.5	0.6	0.8	1.0	1.1	1.2	1.3	1.4
15-19 mo	0.9452	0.7070	0.39409	0.1	0.2	0.3	0.4	0.5	0.7	0.9	1.0	1.2	1.2	1.4
16-20 mo	0.9480	0.6637	0.41387	0.1	0.2	0.2	0.4	0.5	0.7	0.9	1.0	1.1	1.2	1.3
17-21 mo	0.9500	0.6277	0.43237	0.0	0.1	0.2	0.4	0.4	0.6	0.8	0.9	1.1	1.1	1.3
18-22 mo	0.9518	0.5923	0.45102	0.0	0.1	0.2	0.3	0.4	0.6	0.8	0.9	1.0	1.1	1.2
19-23 mo	0.9535	0.5575	0.46942	0.0	0.1	0.1	0.3	0.4	0.6	0.7	0.8	1.0	1.1	1.2
20-24 mo	0.9550	0.5248	0.48711	0.0	0.1	0.1	0.3	0.4	0.5	0.7	0.8	1.0	1.0	1.1

Table 30   Boys 4-month head circumference increments (cm) - *continued*

Interval	L	M	S	-3SD	-2SD	-1SD	Median	+1SD	+2SD	+3SD
0-4 mo	0.3279	7.1133	0.12440	4.8	5.5	6.3	7.1	8.0	9.0	10.1
1-5 mo	0.4212	5.4806	0.12713	3.6	4.2	4.8	5.5	6.2	7.0	7.8
2-6 mo	0.5076	4.2702	0.13454	2.7	3.2	3.7	4.3	4.9	5.5	6.2
3-7 mo	0.5840	3.5185	0.14592	2.1	2.6	3.0	3.5	4.0	4.6	5.2
4-8 mo	0.6557	2.9255	0.16106	1.6	2.0	2.5	2.9	3.4	3.9	4.5
5-9 mo	0.7179	2.4506	0.17841	1.2	1.6	2.0	2.5	2.9	3.4	3.9
6-10 mo	0.7719	2.0780	0.19784	0.9	1.3	1.7	2.1	2.5	2.9	3.4
7-11 mo	0.8180	1.7696	0.21918	0.7	1.0	1.4	1.8	2.2	2.6	3.0
8-12 mo	0.8532	1.5301	0.24082	0.5	0.8	1.2	1.5	1.9	2.3	2.7
9-13 mo	0.8808	1.3368	0.26394	0.3	0.7	1.0	1.3	1.7	2.1	2.4
10-14 mo	0.9009	1.1844	0.28656	0.2	0.5	0.9	1.2	1.5	1.9	2.2
11-15 mo	0.9166	1.0457	0.30970	0.1	0.4	0.7	1.0	1.4	1.7	2.0
12-16 mo	0.9278	0.9301	0.33162	0.1	0.3	0.6	0.9	1.2	1.6	1.9
13-17 mo	0.9357	0.8359	0.35292	0.0	0.3	0.5	0.8	1.1	1.4	1.7
14-18 mo	0.9414	0.7605	0.37421	0.0	0.2	0.5	0.8	1.0	1.3	1.6
15-19 mo	0.9452	0.7070	0.39409	0.0	0.2	0.4	0.7	1.0	1.3	1.6
16-20 mo	0.9480	0.6637	0.41387	0.0	0.1	0.4	0.7	0.9	1.2	1.5
17-21 mo	0.9500	0.6277	0.43237	0.0	0.1	0.4	0.6	0.9	1.2	1.5
18-22 mo	0.9518	0.5923	0.45102	0.0	0.1	0.3	0.6	0.9	1.1	1.4
19-23 mo	0.9535	0.5575	0.46942	0.0	0.1	0.3	0.6	0.8	1.1	1.4
20-24 mo	0.9550	0.5248	0.48711	0.0	0.0	0.3	0.5	0.8	1.0	1.3

Table 31 Girls 4-month head circumference increments (cm)

Interval	L	M	S	1st	3rd	5th	15th	25th	50th	75th	85th	95th	97th	99th
0-4 mo	0.5215	6.6605	0.12888	4.8	5.1	5.3	5.8	6.1	6.7	7.3	7.6	8.1	8.4	8.8
1-5 mo	0.5902	5.0750	0.13444	3.6	3.9	4.0	4.4	4.6	5.1	5.5	5.8	6.2	6.4	6.8
2-6 mo	0.6469	4.0154	0.14318	2.8	3.0	3.1	3.4	3.6	4.0	4.4	4.6	5.0	5.1	5.4
3-7 mo	0.6952	3.3542	0.15397	2.2	2.4	2.5	2.8	3.0	3.4	3.7	3.9	4.2	4.4	4.6
4-8 mo	0.7374	2.8419	0.16676	1.8	2.0	2.1	2.4	2.5	2.8	3.2	3.3	3.6	3.8	4.0
5-9 mo	0.7748	2.3945	0.18192	1.4	1.6	1.7	2.0	2.1	2.4	2.7	2.9	3.1	3.2	3.5
6-10 mo	0.8085	2.0271	0.19915	1.1	1.3	1.4	1.6	1.8	2.0	2.3	2.5	2.7	2.8	3.0
7-11 mo	0.8391	1.7353	0.21812	0.9	1.0	1.1	1.4	1.5	1.7	2.0	2.1	2.4	2.5	2.6
8-12 mo	0.8672	1.5073	0.23888	0.7	0.9	0.9	1.1	1.3	1.5	1.8	1.9	2.1	2.2	2.4
9-13 mo	0.8931	1.3296	0.26147	0.6	0.7	0.8	1.0	1.1	1.3	1.6	1.7	1.9	2.0	2.2
10-14 mo	0.9172	1.1864	0.28575	0.4	0.6	0.6	0.8	1.0	1.2	1.4	1.5	1.8	1.8	2.0
11-15 mo	0.9397	1.0642	0.31149	0.3	0.5	0.5	0.7	0.8	1.1	1.3	1.4	1.6	1.7	1.8
12-16 mo	0.9608	0.9573	0.33813	0.2	0.4	0.4	0.6	0.7	1.0	1.2	1.3	1.5	1.6	1.7
13-17 mo	0.9808	0.8664	0.36514	0.1	0.3	0.3	0.5	0.7	0.9	1.1	1.2	1.4	1.5	1.6
14-18 mo	0.9996	0.7940	0.39238	0.1	0.2	0.3	0.5	0.6	0.8	1.0	1.1	1.3	1.4	1.5
15-19 mo	1.0175	0.7411	0.41976	0.0	0.1	0.2	0.4	0.5	0.7	1.0	1.1	1.3	1.3	1.5
16-20 mo	1.0344	0.6953	0.44691	0.0	0.1	0.2	0.4	0.5	0.7	0.9	1.0	1.2	1.3	1.4
17-21 mo	1.0506	0.6457	0.47350	0.0	0.0	0.1	0.3	0.4	0.6	0.9	1.0	1.1	1.2	1.3
18-22 mo	1.0661	0.5953	0.49958	0.0	0.0	0.1	0.3	0.4	0.6	0.8	0.9	1.1	1.1	1.3
19-23 mo	1.0810	0.5473	0.52538	0.0	0.0	0.0	0.2	0.4	0.5	0.7	0.8	1.0	1.1	1.2
20-24 mo	1.0952	0.5013	0.55112	0.0	0.0	0.0	0.2	0.3	0.5	0.7	0.8	0.9	1.0	1.1

Table 31 Girls 4-month head circumference increments (cm) - *continued*

Interval	L	M	S	-3SD	-2SD	-1SD	Median	+1SD	+2SD	+3SD
0-4 mo	0.5215	6.6605	0.12888	4.3	5.0	5.8	6.7	7.5	8.5	9.5
1-5 mo	0.5902	5.0750	0.13444	3.2	3.8	4.4	5.1	5.8	6.5	7.3
2-6 mo	0.6469	4.0154	0.14318	2.4	2.9	3.5	4.0	4.6	5.2	5.9
3-7 mo	0.6952	3.3542	0.15397	1.9	2.4	2.9	3.4	3.9	4.4	5.0
4-8 mo	0.7374	2.8419	0.16676	1.5	1.9	2.4	2.8	3.3	3.8	4.4
5-9 mo	0.7748	2.3945	0.18192	1.2	1.6	2.0	2.4	2.8	3.3	3.8
6-10 mo	0.8085	2.0271	0.19915	0.9	1.3	1.6	2.0	2.4	2.9	3.3
7-11 mo	0.8391	1.7353	0.21812	0.7	1.0	1.4	1.7	2.1	2.5	2.9
8-12 mo	0.8672	1.5073	0.23888	0.5	0.8	1.2	1.5	1.9	2.2	2.6
9-13 mo	0.8931	1.3296	0.26147	0.3	0.7	1.0	1.3	1.7	2.0	2.4
10-14 mo	0.9172	1.1864	0.28575	0.2	0.5	0.9	1.2	1.5	1.9	2.2
11-15 mo	0.9397	1.0642	0.31149	0.1	0.4	0.7	1.1	1.4	1.7	2.1
12-16 mo	0.9608	0.9573	0.33813	0.0	0.3	0.6	1.0	1.3	1.6	1.9
13-17 mo	0.9808	0.8664	0.36514	0.0	0.2	0.6	0.9	1.2	1.5	1.8
14-18 mo	0.9996	0.7940	0.39238	0.0	0.2	0.5	0.8	1.1	1.4	1.7
15-19 mo	1.0175	0.7411	0.41976	0.0	0.1	0.4	0.7	1.1	1.4	1.7
16-20 mo	1.0344	0.6953	0.44691	0.0	0.1	0.4	0.7	1.0	1.3	1.6
17-21 mo	1.0506	0.6457	0.47350	0.0	0.0	0.3	0.6	0.9	1.2	1.5
18-22 mo	1.0661	0.5953	0.49958	0.0	0.0	0.3	0.6	0.9	1.2	1.5
19-23 mo	1.0810	0.5473	0.52538	0.0	0.0	0.3	0.5	0.8	1.1	1.4
20-24 mo	1.0952	0.5013	0.55112	0.0	0.0	0.2	0.5	0.8	1.0	1.3

Table 32 Boys 6-month head circumference increments (cm)

Interval	L	M	S	1st	3rd	5th	15th	25th	50th	75th	85th	95th	97th	99th
0-6 mo	0.4441	8.8640	0.11010	6.8	7.1	7.3	7.9	8.2	8.9	9.5	9.9	10.6	10.8	11.3
1-7 mo	0.4988	6.9439	0.11688	5.2	5.5	5.7	6.1	6.4	6.9	7.5	7.8	8.3	8.6	9.0
2-8 mo	0.5465	5.5066	0.12498	4.0	4.3	4.4	4.8	5.1	5.5	6.0	6.2	6.7	6.9	7.2
3-9 mo	0.5888	4.5260	0.13512	3.2	3.4	3.6	3.9	4.1	4.5	4.9	5.2	5.6	5.7	6.0
4-10 mo	0.6269	3.7983	0.14708	2.6	2.8	2.9	3.2	3.4	3.8	4.2	4.4	4.8	4.9	5.2
5-11 mo	0.6616	3.2122	0.16026	2.1	2.3	2.4	2.7	2.9	3.2	3.6	3.8	4.1	4.2	4.5
6-12 mo	0.6933	2.7354	0.17427	1.7	1.9	2.0	2.3	2.4	2.7	3.1	3.2	3.6	3.7	3.9
7-13 mo	0.7226	2.3511	0.18884	1.4	1.6	1.7	1.9	2.1	2.4	2.7	2.8	3.1	3.2	3.4
8-14 mo	0.7499	2.0461	0.20363	1.1	1.3	1.4	1.6	1.8	2.0	2.3	2.5	2.8	2.9	3.1
9-15 mo	0.7754	1.7985	0.21837	0.9	1.1	1.2	1.4	1.5	1.8	2.1	2.2	2.5	2.6	2.8
10-16 mo	0.7993	1.5932	0.23280	0.8	0.9	1.0	1.2	1.3	1.6	1.8	2.0	2.2	2.3	2.5
11-17 mo	0.8218	1.4211	0.24672	0.7	0.8	0.9	1.1	1.2	1.4	1.7	1.8	2.0	2.1	2.3
12-18 mo	0.8431	1.2795	0.26021	0.5	0.7	0.8	0.9	1.1	1.3	1.5	1.6	1.8	1.9	2.1
13-19 mo	0.8633	1.1676	0.27339	0.5	0.6	0.7	0.8	1.0	1.2	1.4	1.5	1.7	1.8	1.9
14-20 mo	0.8825	1.0785	0.28632	0.4	0.5	0.6	0.8	0.9	1.1	1.3	1.4	1.6	1.7	1.8
15-21 mo	0.9009	1.0078	0.29903	0.3	0.5	0.5	0.7	0.8	1.0	1.2	1.3	1.5	1.6	1.7
16-22 mo	0.9184	0.9483	0.31159	0.3	0.4	0.5	0.6	0.8	0.9	1.1	1.3	1.4	1.5	1.7
17-23 mo	0.9351	0.8976	0.32406	0.2	0.4	0.4	0.6	0.7	0.9	1.1	1.2	1.4	1.5	1.6
18-24 mo	0.9512	0.8511	0.33648	0.2	0.3	0.4	0.6	0.7	0.9	1.0	1.2	1.3	1.4	1.5

Table 32 Boys 6-month head circumference increments (cm) - *continued*

Interval	L	M	S	-3SD	-2SD	-1SD	Median	+1SD	+2SD	+3SD
0-6 mo	0.4441	8.8640	0.11010	6.2	7.0	7.9	8.9	9.9	10.9	12.1
1-7 mo	0.4988	6.9439	0.11688	4.7	5.4	6.2	6.9	7.8	8.7	9.6
2-8 mo	0.5465	5.5066	0.12498	3.6	4.2	4.8	5.5	6.2	7.0	7.7
3-9 mo	0.5888	4.5260	0.13512	2.8	3.4	3.9	4.5	5.2	5.8	6.5
4-10 mo	0.6269	3.7983	0.14708	2.3	2.7	3.3	3.8	4.4	5.0	5.6
5-11 mo	0.6616	3.2122	0.16026	1.8	2.2	2.7	3.2	3.7	4.3	4.9
6-12 mo	0.6933	2.7354	0.17427	1.4	1.8	2.3	2.7	3.2	3.7	4.3
7-13 mo	0.7226	2.3511	0.18884	1.1	1.5	1.9	2.4	2.8	3.3	3.8
8-14 mo	0.7499	2.0461	0.20363	0.9	1.3	1.6	2.0	2.5	2.9	3.4
9-15 mo	0.7754	1.7985	0.21837	0.7	1.1	1.4	1.8	2.2	2.6	3.1
10-16 mo	0.7993	1.5932	0.23280	0.6	0.9	1.2	1.6	2.0	2.4	2.8
11-17 mo	0.8218	1.4211	0.24672	0.5	0.8	1.1	1.4	1.8	2.2	2.5
12-18 mo	0.8431	1.2795	0.26021	0.4	0.6	1.0	1.3	1.6	2.0	2.3
13-19 mo	0.8633	1.1676	0.27339	0.3	0.6	0.9	1.2	1.5	1.8	2.2
14-20 mo	0.8825	1.0785	0.28632	0.2	0.5	0.8	1.1	1.4	1.7	2.0
15-21 mo	0.9009	1.0078	0.29903	0.2	0.4	0.7	1.0	1.3	1.6	1.9
16-22 mo	0.9184	0.9483	0.31159	0.1	0.4	0.7	0.9	1.2	1.6	1.9
17-23 mo	0.9351	0.8976	0.32406	0.1	0.3	0.6	0.9	1.2	1.5	1.8
18-24 mo	0.9512	0.8511	0.33648	0.0	0.3	0.6	0.9	1.1	1.4	1.7

Table 33   **Girls 6-month head circumference increments (cm)**

Interval	L	M	S	1st	3rd	5th	15th	25th	50th	75th	85th	95th	97th	99th
0-6 mo	0.2608	8.2683	0.11607	6.2	6.6	6.8	7.3	7.6	8.3	8.9	9.3	10.0	10.2	10.7
1-7 mo	0.3426	6.5037	0.11997	4.9	5.1	5.3	5.7	6.0	6.5	7.0	7.3	7.9	8.1	8.5
2-8 mo	0.4140	5.2206	0.12590	3.8	4.1	4.2	4.6	4.8	5.2	5.7	5.9	6.4	6.5	6.9
3-9 mo	0.4774	4.3410	0.13381	3.1	3.3	3.4	3.8	4.0	4.3	4.7	5.0	5.4	5.5	5.8
4-10 mo	0.5344	3.6748	0.14324	2.5	2.7	2.9	3.1	3.3	3.7	4.0	4.2	4.6	4.7	5.0
5-11 mo	0.5863	3.1336	0.15447	2.1	2.3	2.4	2.6	2.8	3.1	3.5	3.7	4.0	4.1	4.3
6-12 mo	0.6338	2.6890	0.16777	1.7	1.9	2.0	2.2	2.4	2.7	3.0	3.2	3.5	3.6	3.8
7-13 mo	0.6777	2.3226	0.18258	1.4	1.6	1.7	1.9	2.0	2.3	2.6	2.8	3.1	3.2	3.4
8-14 mo	0.7186	2.0288	0.19851	1.2	1.3	1.4	1.6	1.8	2.0	2.3	2.5	2.7	2.8	3.0
9-15 mo	0.7567	1.7978	0.21524	1.0	1.1	1.2	1.4	1.5	1.8	2.1	2.2	2.5	2.6	2.7
10-16 mo	0.7925	1.6098	0.23248	0.8	0.9	1.0	1.2	1.4	1.6	1.9	2.0	2.2	2.3	2.5
11-17 mo	0.8262	1.4500	0.24989	0.7	0.8	0.9	1.1	1.2	1.5	1.7	1.8	2.1	2.2	2.3
12-18 mo	0.8581	1.3166	0.26722	0.5	0.7	0.8	1.0	1.1	1.3	1.6	1.7	1.9	2.0	2.2
13-19 mo	0.8884	1.2111	0.28419	0.4	0.6	0.7	0.9	1.0	1.2	1.4	1.6	1.8	1.9	2.0
14-20 mo	0.9172	1.1249	0.30032	0.4	0.5	0.6	0.8	0.9	1.1	1.4	1.5	1.7	1.8	1.9
15-21 mo	0.9446	1.0506	0.31516	0.3	0.4	0.5	0.7	0.8	1.1	1.3	1.4	1.6	1.7	1.8
16-22 mo	0.9708	0.9819	0.32846	0.2	0.4	0.5	0.6	0.8	1.0	1.2	1.3	1.5	1.6	1.7
17-23 mo	0.9959	0.9149	0.34024	0.2	0.3	0.4	0.6	0.7	0.9	1.1	1.2	1.4	1.5	1.6
18-24 mo	1.0200	0.8494	0.35116	0.1	0.3	0.4	0.5	0.6	0.8	1.1	1.2	1.3	1.4	1.5

Table 33   Girls 6-month head circumference increments (cm) - *continued*

Interval	L	M	S	-3SD	-2SD	-1SD	Median	+1SD	+2SD	+3SD
0-6 mo	0.2608	8.2683	0.11607	5.7	6.5	7.3	8.3	9.3	10.4	11.5
1-7 mo	0.3426	6.5037	0.11997	4.4	5.1	5.8	6.5	7.3	8.2	9.1
2-8 mo	0.4140	5.2206	0.12590	3.5	4.0	4.6	5.2	5.9	6.6	7.4
3-9 mo	0.4774	4.3410	0.13381	2.8	3.3	3.8	4.3	4.9	5.6	6.3
4-10 mo	0.5344	3.6748	0.14324	2.3	2.7	3.2	3.7	4.2	4.8	5.4
5-11 mo	0.5863	3.1336	0.15447	1.8	2.2	2.7	3.1	3.6	4.2	4.7
6-12 mo	0.6338	2.6890	0.16777	1.5	1.8	2.3	2.7	3.2	3.6	4.2
7-13 mo	0.6777	2.3226	0.18258	1.2	1.5	1.9	2.3	2.8	3.2	3.7
8-14 mo	0.7186	2.0288	0.19851	0.9	1.3	1.6	2.0	2.4	2.9	3.3
9-15 mo	0.7567	1.7978	0.21524	0.7	1.1	1.4	1.8	2.2	2.6	3.0
10-16 mo	0.7925	1.6098	0.23248	0.6	0.9	1.2	1.6	2.0	2.4	2.8
11-17 mo	0.8262	1.4500	0.24989	0.5	0.8	1.1	1.5	1.8	2.2	2.6
12-18 mo	0.8581	1.3166	0.26722	0.3	0.6	1.0	1.3	1.7	2.0	2.4
13-19 mo	0.8884	1.2111	0.28419	0.2	0.5	0.9	1.2	1.6	1.9	2.3
14-20 mo	0.9172	1.1249	0.30032	0.2	0.5	0.8	1.1	1.5	1.8	2.2
15-21 mo	0.9446	1.0506	0.31516	0.1	0.4	0.7	1.1	1.4	1.7	2.1
16-22 mo	0.9708	0.9819	0.32846	0.0	0.3	0.7	1.0	1.3	1.6	2.0
17-23 mo	0.9959	0.9149	0.34024	0.0	0.3	0.6	0.9	1.2	1.5	1.9
18-24 mo	1.0200	0.8494	0.35116	0.0	0.2	0.5	0.8	1.1	1.4	1.7

Appendix A5 Diagnostics

A5.1a 2-month intervals for boys

Table A5.1   Q-test for z-scores from selected model [BCPE(x=age$^{0.05}$, df(μ)=8, df(σ)=4, df(ν)=4, τ=2)] for 2-month head circumference velocity for boys

Age (days)	Group	N	z1	z2	z3
55 to 76	**0-2 mo**	423	0.2	1.2	-0.9
76 to 107	**1-3 mo**	416	0.4	-0.3	1.1
107 to 137	**2-4 mo**	415	-1.3	-0.5	1.5
137 to 168	**3-5 mo**	413	1.3	-1.4	0.2
168 to 198	**4-6 mo**	415	0.1	-0.7	-0.9
198 to 229	**5-7 mo**	412	-0.5	1.0	-0.1
229 to 259	**6-8 mo**	416	0.7	0.1	0.6
259 to 289	**7-9 mo**	407	-1.0	-0.8	2.2
289 to 320	**8-10 mo**	403	-0.4	1.5	-1.8
320 to 350	**9-11 mo**	409	0.9	0.0	-0.7
350 to 396	**10-12 mo**	404	-0.6	0.3	-1.0
396 to 433	**12-14 mo**	414	-0.6	1.5	-1.1
Overall Q stats		4947	6.9	10.5	16.2
degrees of freedom			4.0	9.5	8.0
p-value			0.1419	0.3574	0.0403

Note: Absolute values of z1, z2 or z3 larger than 2 indicate misfit of, respectively, mean, variance or skewness.

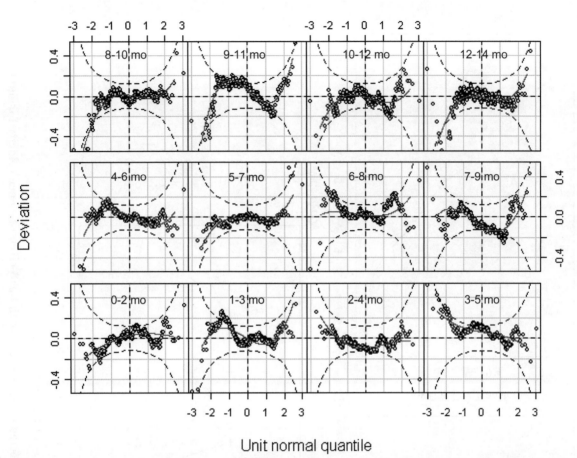

Figure A5.1 Worm plots from selected model [BCPE(x=age$^{0.05}$, df(μ)=8, df(σ)=4, df(ν)=4, τ=2)] for 2-month head circumference velocity for boys

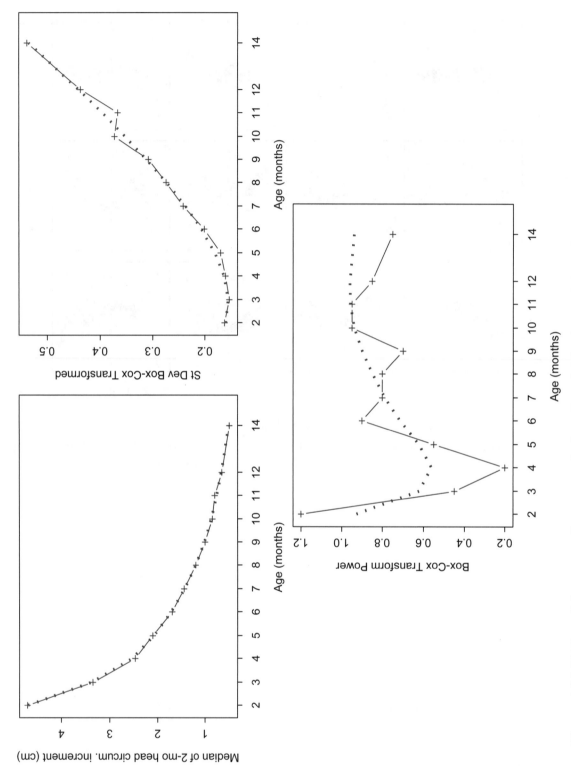

Figure A5.2 Fitting of the μ, σ, and ν curves of selected model for 2-month head circumference velocity for boys

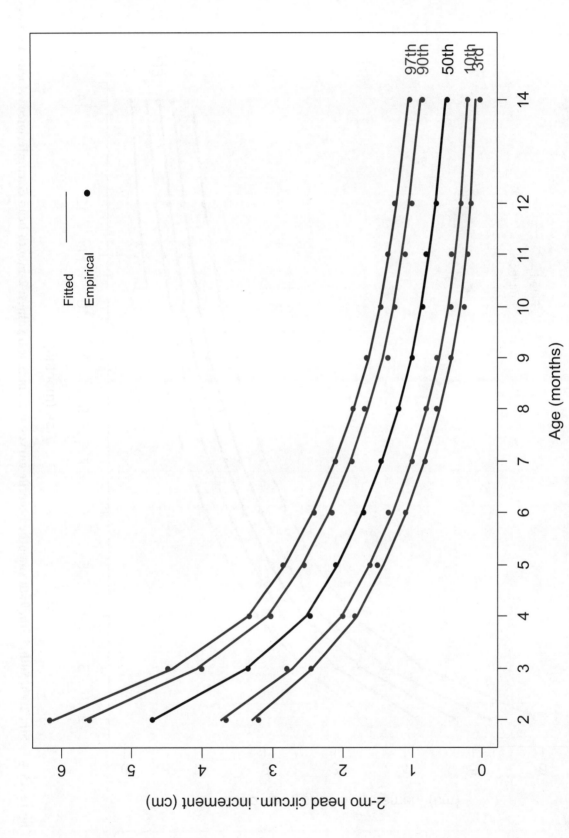

Figure A5.3 3rd, 10th, 50th, 90th, 97th smoothed centile curves and empirical values: 2-month head circumference velocity for boys

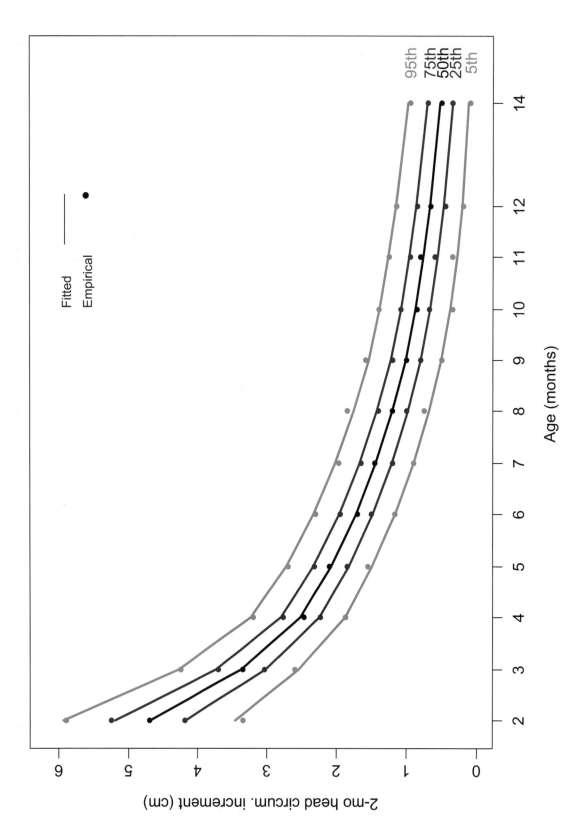

Figure A5.4   5th, 25th, 50th, 75th, 95th smoothed centile curves and empirical values: 2-month head circumference velocity for boys

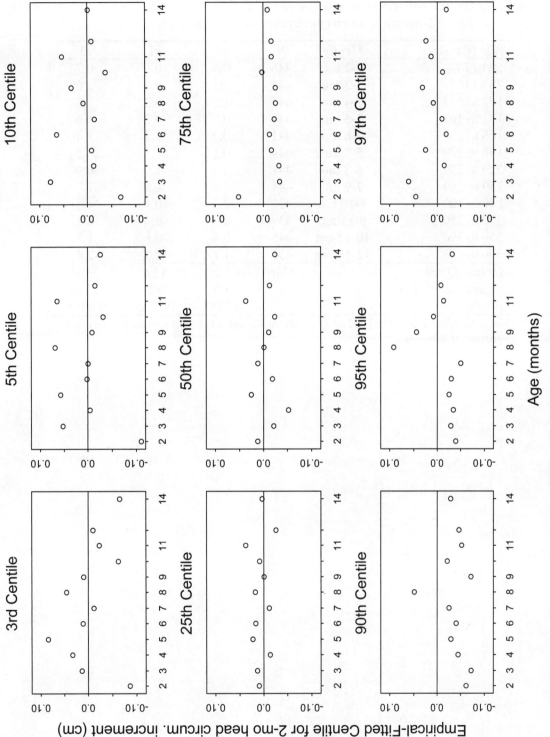

Figure A5.5 Centile residuals from fitting selected model for 2-month head circumference velocity for boys

A5.1b 2-month intervals for girls

Table A5.2   **Q-test for z-scores from selected model [BCPE(x=age$^{0.05}$, df(μ)=8, df(σ)=4, df(ν)=1, τ=2)] for 2-month head circumference velocity for girls**

Age (days)	Group	N	z1	z2	z3
58 to 76	**0-2 mo**	446	0.4	0.9	-0.7
76 to 107	**1-3 mo**	443	0.1	-0.4	1.0
107 to 137	**2-4 mo**	441	-1.1	-0.2	1.9
137 to 168	**3-5 mo**	444	0.7	-0.2	1.6
168 to 198	**4-6 mo**	441	0.2	0.3	1.4
198 to 229	**5-7 mo**	444	0.1	-1.1	0.2
229 to 259	**6-8 mo**	441	0.7	-1.0	-0.9
259 to 289	**7-9 mo**	444	-0.9	1.8	1.7
289 to 320	**8-10 mo**	437	-0.7	0.1	-1.3
320 to 350	**9-11 mo**	439	0.3	0.6	-2.7
350 to 396	**10-12 mo**	445	0.4	-0.6	1.7
396 to 433	**12-14 mo**	451	-1.1	2.3	-2.4
Overall Q stats		5316	5.1	12.4	31.1
degrees of freedom			4.0	9.5	11.0
p-value			0.2737	0.2255	0.0011

Note: Absolute values of z1, z2 or z3 larger than 2 indicate misfit of, respectively, mean, variance or skewness.

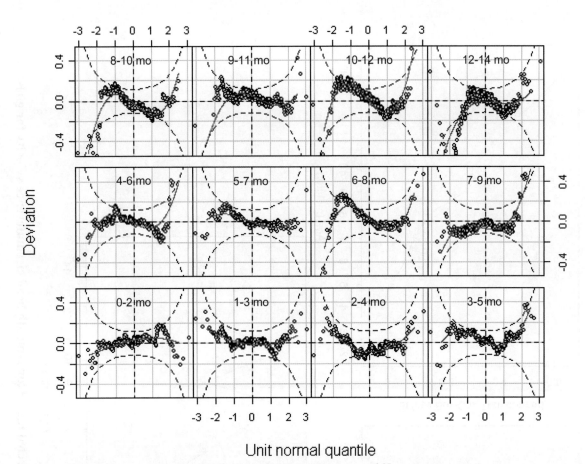

Figure A5.6 Worm plots from selected model [BCPE(x=age$^{0.05}$, df(μ)=8, df(σ)=4, df(ν)=1, τ=2)] for 2-month head circumference velocity for girls

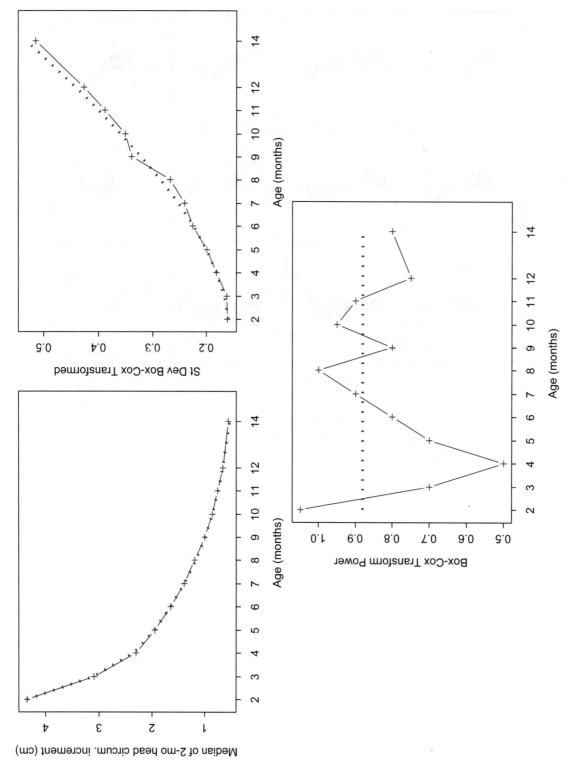

Figure A5.7 Fitting of the μ, σ, and ν curves of selected model for 2-month head circumference velocity for girls

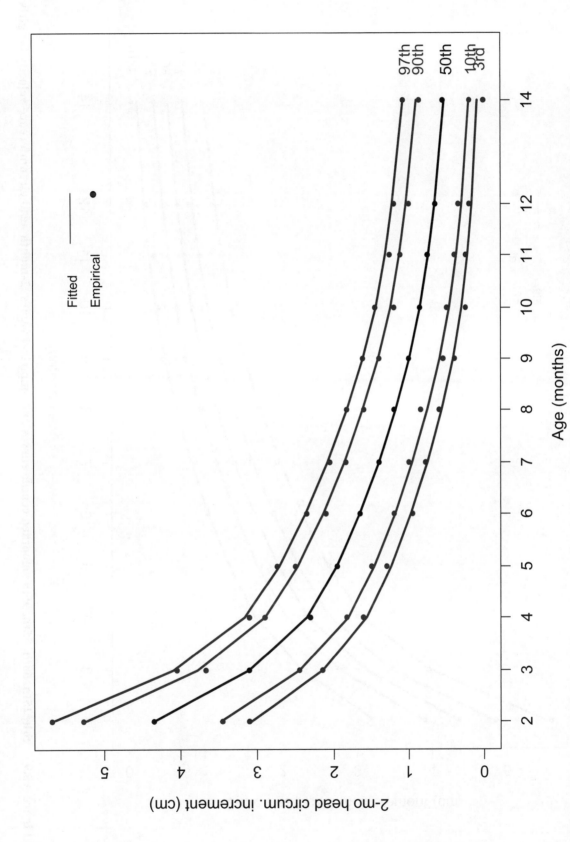

Figure A5.8   3rd, 10th, 50th, 90th, 97th smoothed centile curves and empirical values: 2-month head circumference velocity for girls

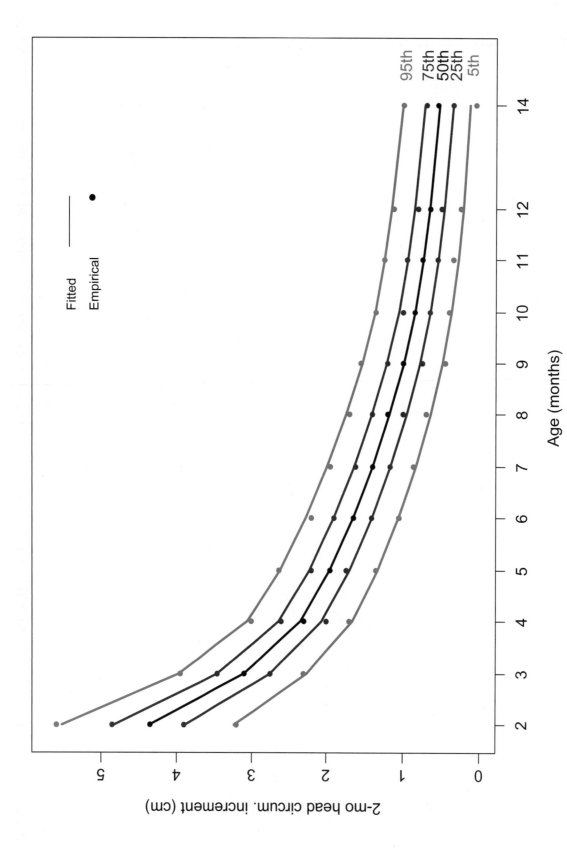

Figure A5.9   5th, 25th, 50th, 75th, 95th smoothed centile curves and empirical values: 2-month head circumference velocity for girls

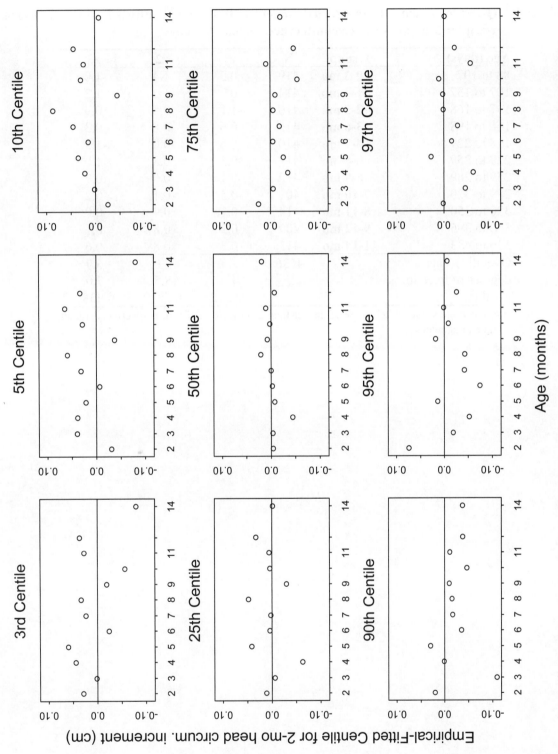

Figure A5.10 Centile residuals from fitting selected model for 2-month head circumference velocity for girls

A5.2a 3-month intervals for boys

Table A5.3   **Q-test for z-scores from selected model [BCPE(x=age$^{0.05}$, df(μ)=7, df(σ)=4, df(ν)=4, τ=2)] for 3-month head circumference velocity for boys**

Age (days)	Group	N	z1	z2	z3
88 to 107	**0-3 mo**	419	0.5	1.4	-1.0
107 to 137	**1-4 mo**	414	0.2	-1.2	1.2
137 to 168	**2-5 mo**	416	-1.1	-0.5	0.9
168 to 198	**3-6 mo**	416	0.6	-0.8	0.3
198 to 229	**4-7 mo**	410	0.5	0.0	-1.3
229 to 259	**5-8 mo**	412	-0.3	0.8	1.0
259 to 289	**6-9 mo**	410	-0.1	0.0	0.7
289 to 320	**7-10 mo**	403	-0.5	-0.1	0.2
320 to 350	**8-11 mo**	414	0.1	0.9	0.0
350 to 396	**9-12 mo**	409	0.2	-0.8	0.1
396 to 433	**11-14 mo**	413	-0.3	0.8	-0.6
Overall Q stats		4536	2.5	7.0	6.9
degrees of freedom			4.0	8.5	7.0
p-value			0.6375	0.5872	0.4380

Note: Absolute values of z1, z2 or z3 larger than 2 indicate misfit of, respectively, mean, variance or skewness.

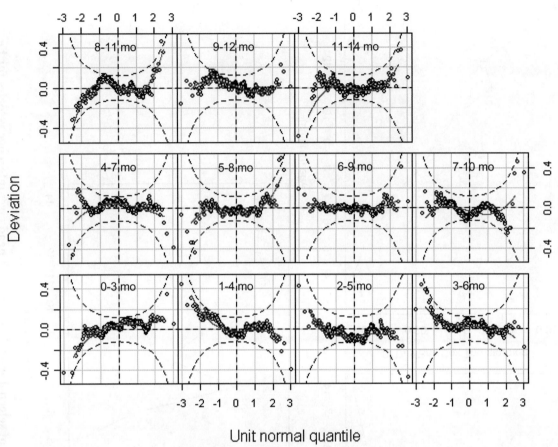

Figure A5.11 Worm plots from selected model [BCPE(x=age$^{0.05}$, df(μ)=7, df(σ)=4, df(ν)=4, τ=2)] for 3-month head circumference velocity for boys

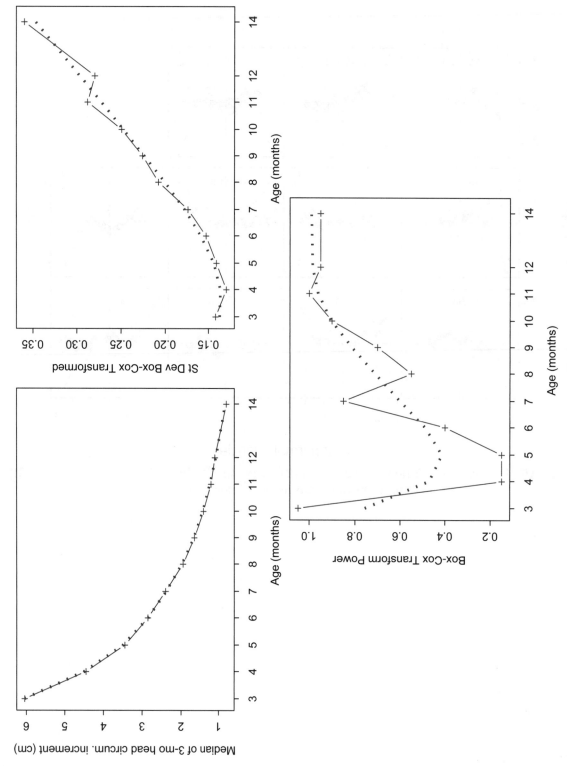

Figure A5.12 Fitting of the μ, σ, and ν curves of selected model for 3-month head circumference velocity for boys

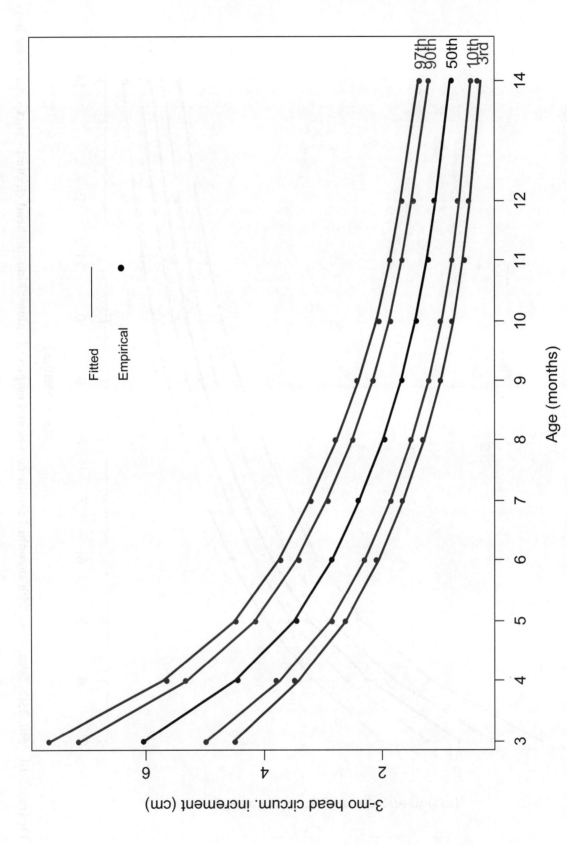

Figure A5.13 3rd, 10th, 50th, 90th, 97th smoothed centile curves and empirical values: 3-month head circumference velocity for boys

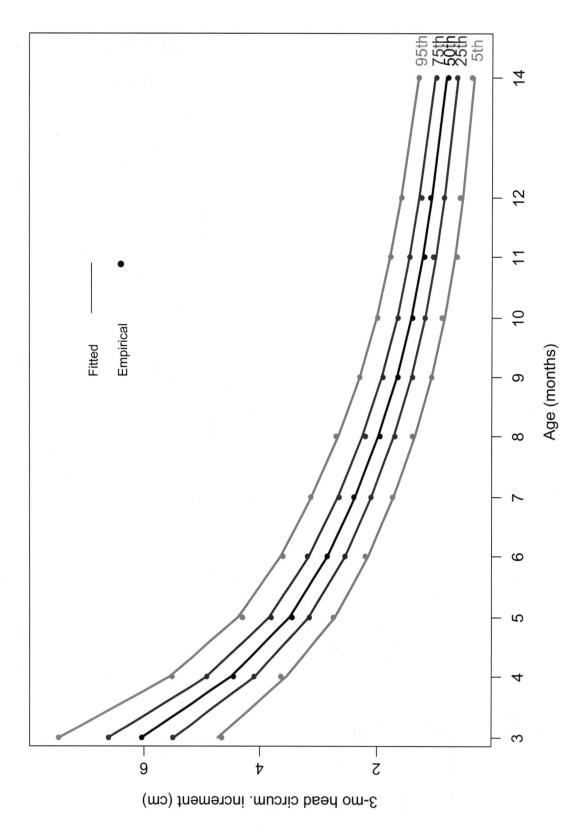

Figure A5.14   5th, 25th, 50th, 75th, 95th smoothed centile curves and empirical values: 3-month head circumference velocity for boys

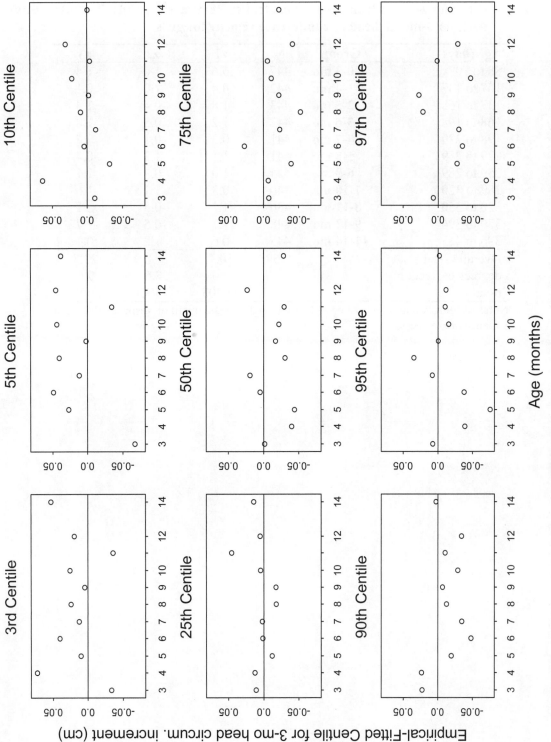

Figure A5.15 Centile residuals from fitting selected model for 3-month head circumference velocity for boys

A5.2b 3-month intervals for girls

Table A5.4   **Q-test for z-scores from selected model [BCPE(x=age$^{0.05}$, df(μ)=7, df(σ)=4, df(ν)=2, τ=2)] for 3-month head circumference velocity for girls**

Age (days)	Group	N	z1	z2	z3
88 to 107	**0-3 mo**	447	0.6	1.0	-1.4
107 to 137	**1-4 mo**	442	0.4	-1.0	0.1
137 to 168	**2-5 mo**	443	-1.8	-0.4	1.4
168 to 198	**3-6 mo**	442	1.2	0.5	1.8
198 to 229	**4-7 mo**	441	-0.3	-0.1	0.7
229 to 259	**5-8 mo**	441	1.1	-1.3	-0.4
259 to 289	**6-9 mo**	444	-1.0	0.7	1.1
289 to 320	**7-10 mo**	440	0.3	1.1	-1.6
320 to 350	**8-11 mo**	436	-1.2	-0.5	2.1
350 to 396	**9-12 mo**	448	1.1	-0.5	-2.7
396 to 433	**11-14 mo**	445	-0.6	1.2	0.4
Overall Q stats		4869	10.7	7.8	23.5
degrees of freedom			4.0	8.5	9.0
p-value			0.0303	0.5067	0.0052

Note: Absolute values of z1, z2 or z3 larger than 2 indicate misfit of, respectively, mean, variance or skewness.

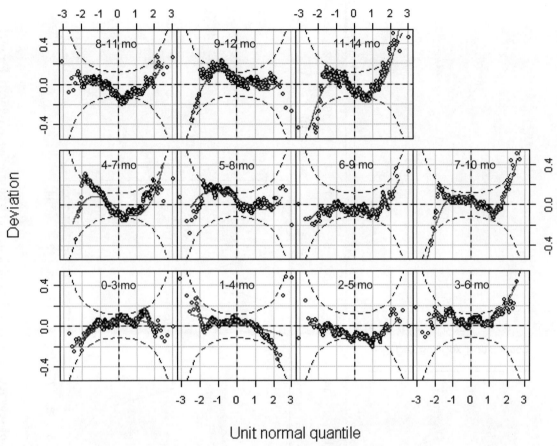

Figure A5.16 Worm plots from selected model [BCPE(x=age$^{0.05}$, df(μ)=7, df(σ)=4, df(ν)=2, τ=2)] for 3-month head circumference velocity for girls

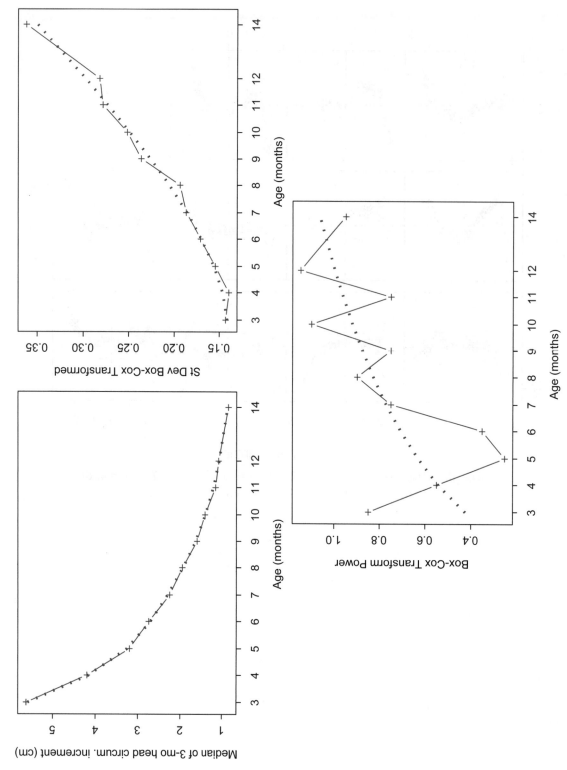

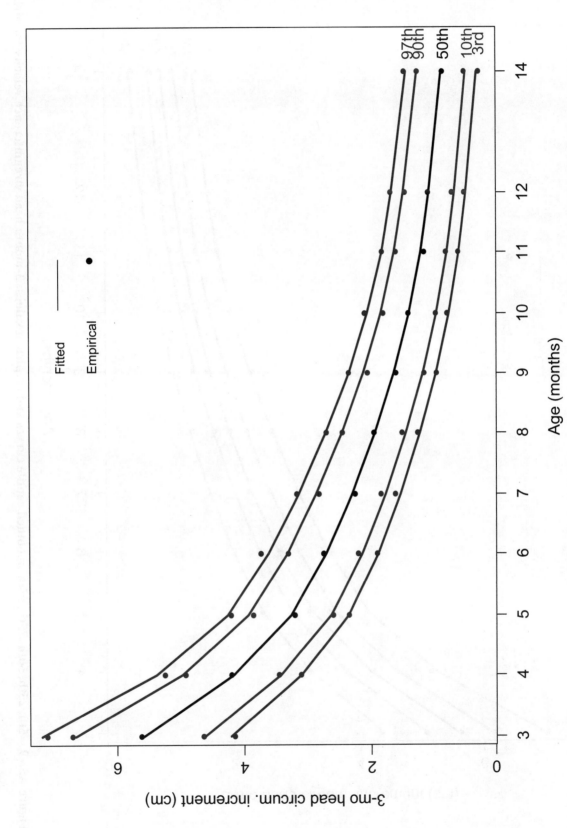

Figure A5.18 3rd, 10th, 50th, 90th, 97th smoothed centile curves and empirical values: 3-month head circumference velocity for girls

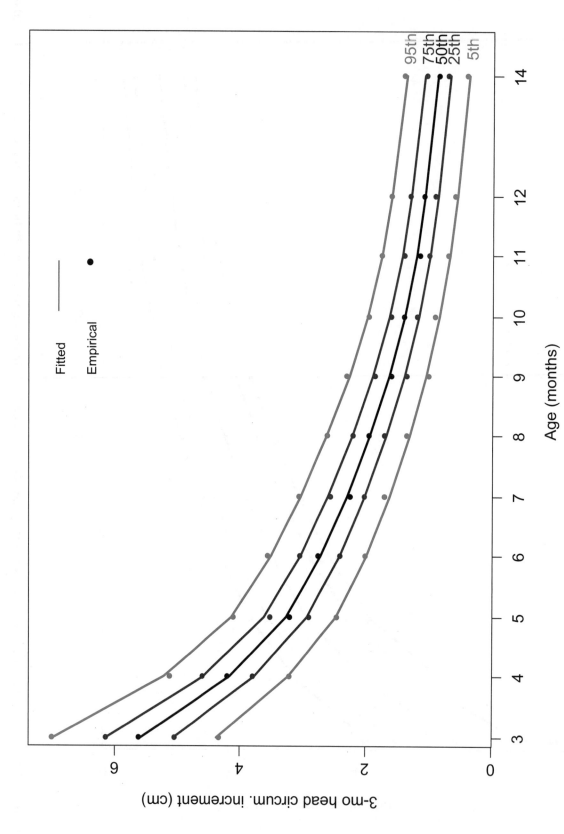

Figure A5.19   5th, 25th, 50th, 75th, 95th smoothed centile curves and empirical values: 3-month head circumference velocity for girls

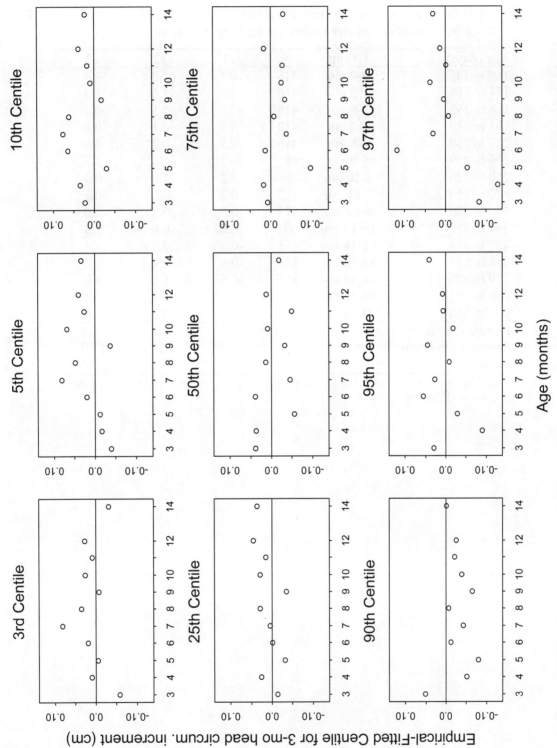

Figure A5.20 Centile residuals from fitting selected model for 3-month head circumference velocity for girls

A5.3a 4-month intervals for boys

Table A5.5   Q-test for z-scores from selected model [BCPE(x=age$^{0.05}$, df(μ)=10, df(σ)=5, df(ν)=3, τ=2)] for 4-month head circumference velocity for boys

Age (days)	Group	N	z1	z2	z3
119 to 137	**0-4 mo**	418	0.7	1.2	-1.4
137 to 168	**1-5 mo**	416	0.4	-1.0	1.4
168 to 198	**2-6 mo**	419	-1.6	-0.5	0.7
198 to 229	**3-7 mo**	412	0.8	0.1	0.4
229 to 259	**4-8 mo**	410	0.5	-0.2	0.6
259 to 289	**5-9 mo**	407	-0.5	-0.6	1.3
289 to 320	**6-10 mo**	406	0.2	1.0	0.3
320 to 350	**7-11 mo**	412	0.2	-0.5	-0.2
350 to 396	**8-12 mo**	414	-0.5	-0.2	-1.6
396 to 457	**10-14 mo**	402	0.3	0.6	1.3
457 to 518	**12-16 mo**	413	-0.2	0.5	-1.4
518 to 579	**14-18 mo**	409	-0.5	0.4	0.0
579 to 640	**16-20 mo**	415	-0.5	1.5	-1.0
640 to 701	**18-22 mo**	407	0.3	-0.1	-0.4
701 to 750	**20-24 mo**	417	-0.1	0.3	-1.5
Overall Q stats		6177	5.6	7.4	16.4
degrees of freedom			5.0	12.0	12.0
p-value			0.3515	0.8315	0.1724

Note: Absolute values of z1, z2 or z3 larger than 2 indicate misfit of, respectively, mean, variance or skewness.

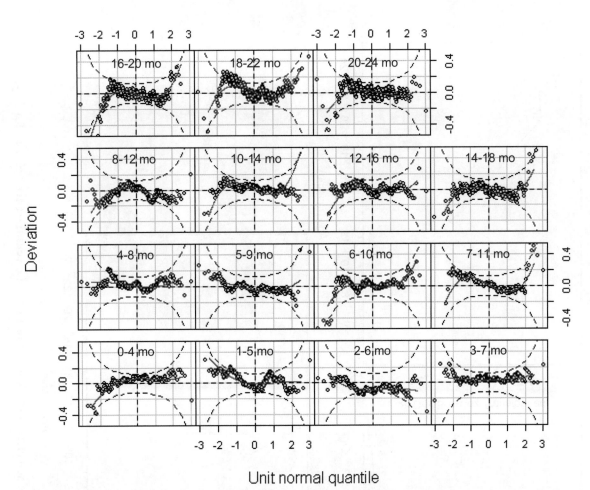

Figure A5.21 Worm plots from selected model [BCPE(x=age$^{0.05}$, df(μ)=10, df(σ)=5, df(ν)=3, τ=2)] for 4-month head circumference velocity for boys

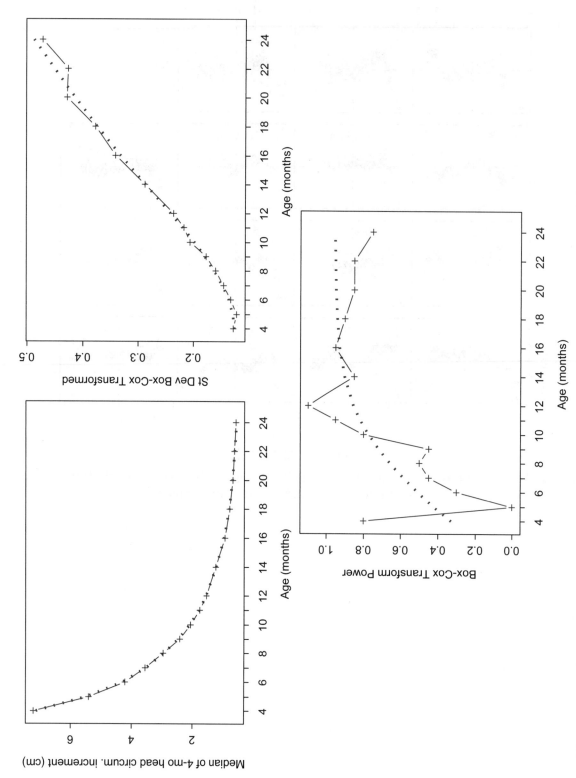

Figure A5.22 Fitting of the μ, σ, and ν curves of selected model for 4-month head circumference velocity for boys

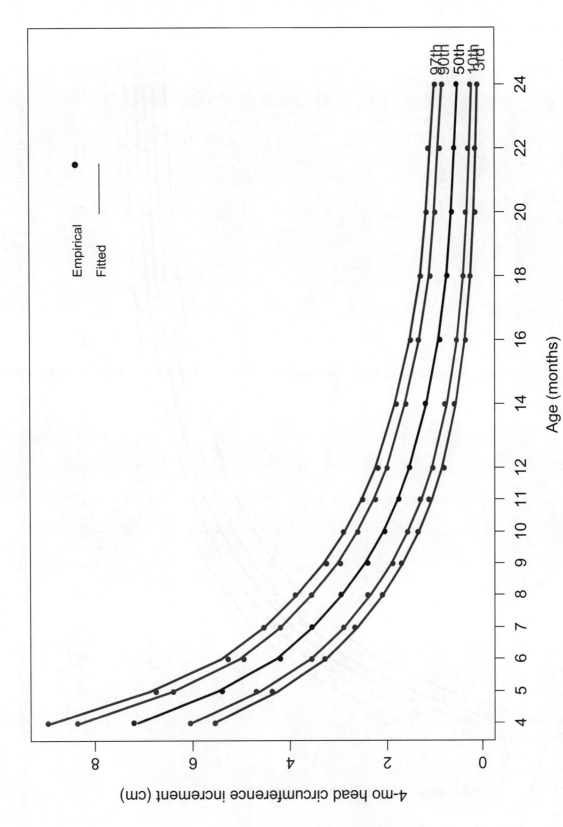

Figure A5.23   3rd, 10th, 50th, 90th, 97th smoothed centile curves and empirical values: 4-month head circumference velocity for boys

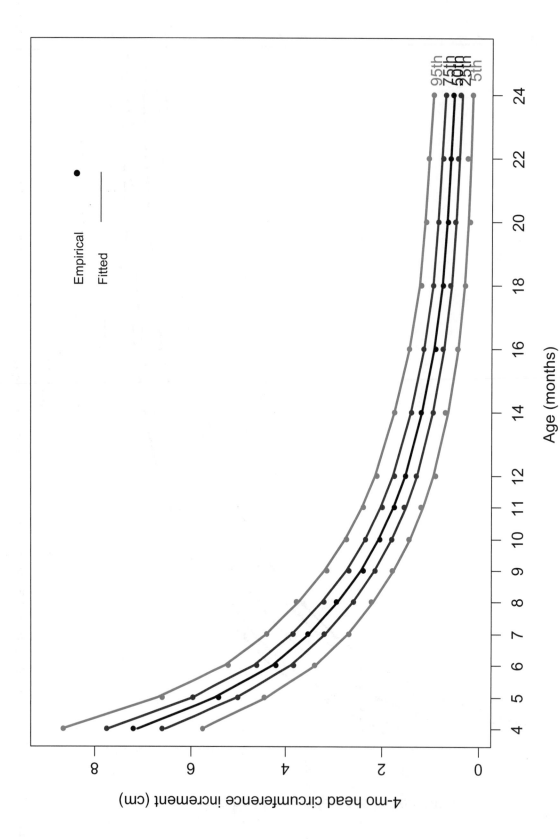

Figure A5.24   5th, 25th, 50th, 75th, 95th smoothed centile curves and empirical values: 4-month head circumference velocity for boys

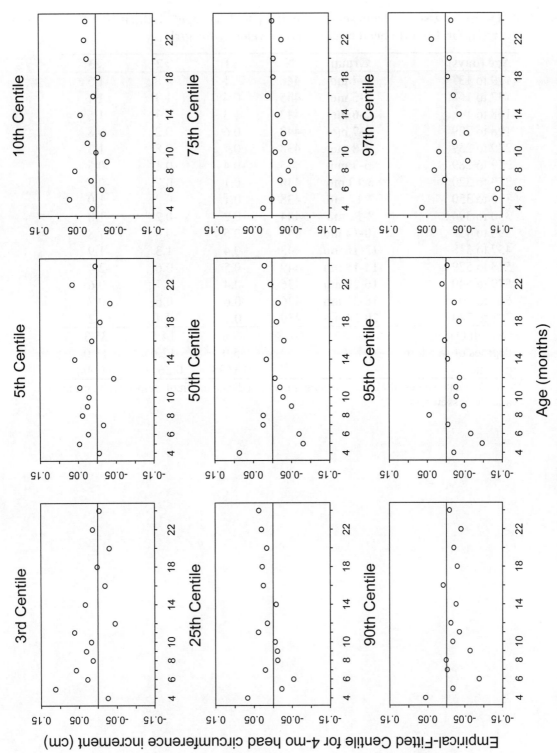

Age (months)

Empirical-Fitted Centile for 4-mo head circumference increment (cm)

Figure A5.25 Centile residuals from fitting selected model for 4-month head circumference velocity for boys

A5.3b 4-month intervals for girls

Table A5.6   Q-test for z-scores from selected model [BCPE(x=age$^{0.05}$, df(μ)=10, df(σ)=5, df(ν)=2, τ=2)] for 4-month head circumference velocity for girls

Age (days)	Group	N	z1	z2	z3
119 to 137	**0-4 mo**	446	1.1	0.8	-1.5
137 to 168	**1-5 mo**	445	-0.4	-1.3	1.1
168 to 198	**2-6 mo**	442	-1.3	0.7	1.5
198 to 229	**3-7 mo**	442	0.6	0.2	0.8
229 to 259	**4-8 mo**	438	0.7	-0.8	1.3
259 to 289	**5-9 mo**	445	-0.4	-0.1	0.5
289 to 320	**6-10 mo**	440	-0.1	0.7	-0.9
320 to 350	**7-11 mo**	438	0.1	-0.2	1.0
350 to 396	**8-12 mo**	444	-0.2	-0.2	-1.0
396 to 457	**10-14 mo**	445	0.5	-0.8	1.8
457 to 518	**12-16 mo**	443	-0.4	1.3	-1.9
518 to 579	**14-18 mo**	449	-0.5	-0.6	-2.4
579 to 640	**16-20 mo**	436	-0.4	2.7	0.6
640 to 701	**18-22 mo**	436	-0.6	0.6	0.7
701 to 749	**20-24 mo**	439	0.7	-0.4	-3.2
Overall Q stats		6628	5.6	14.7	35.3
degrees of freedom			5.0	12.0	13.0
p-value			0.3498	0.2611	0.0008

Note: Absolute values of z1, z2 or z3 larger than 2 indicate misfit of, respectively, mean, variance or skewness.

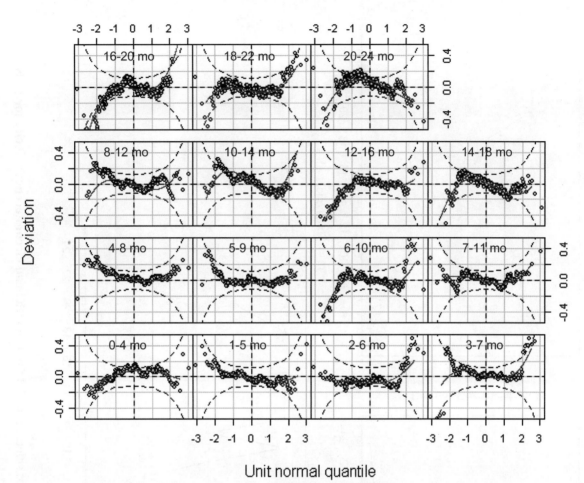

Figure A5.26 Worm plots from selected model [BCPE(x=age$^{0.05}$, df(μ)=10, df(σ)=5, df(ν)=2, τ=2)] for 4-month head circumference velocity for girls

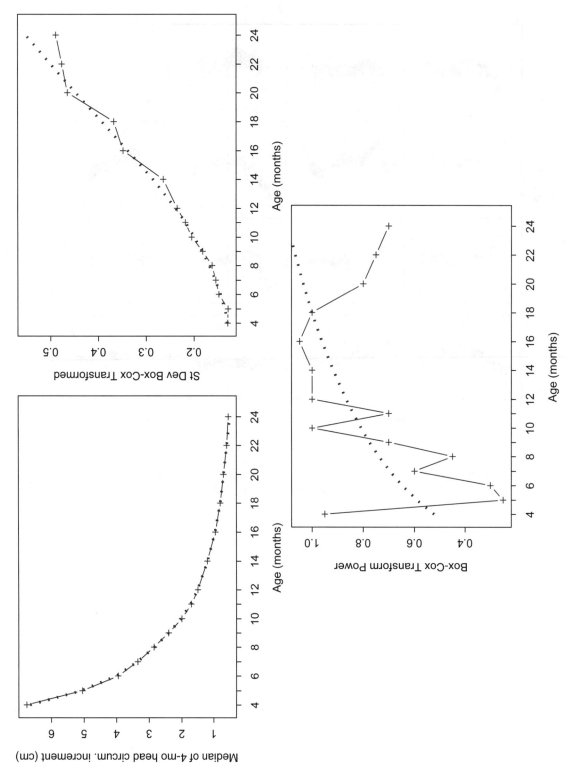

Figure A5.27 Fitting of the μ, σ, and ν curves of selected model for 4-month head circumference velocity for girls

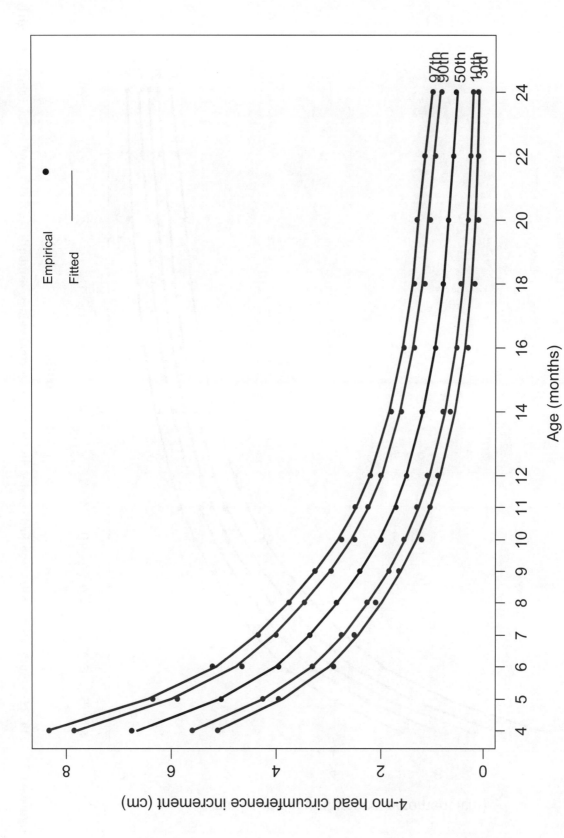

Figure A5.28   3rd, 10th, 50th, 90th, 97th smoothed centile curves and empirical values: 4-month head circumference velocity for girls

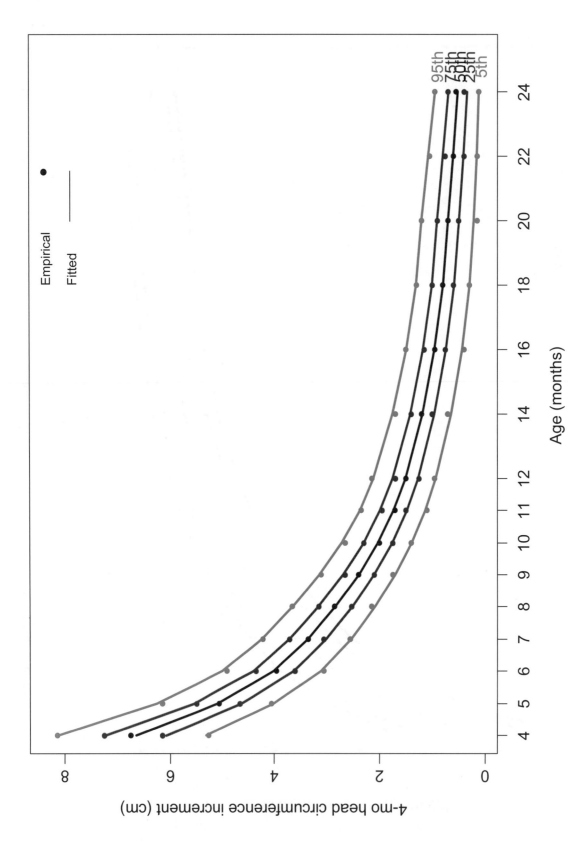

Figure A5.29   5th, 25th, 50th, 75th, 95th smoothed centile curves and empirical values: 4-month head circumference velocity for girls

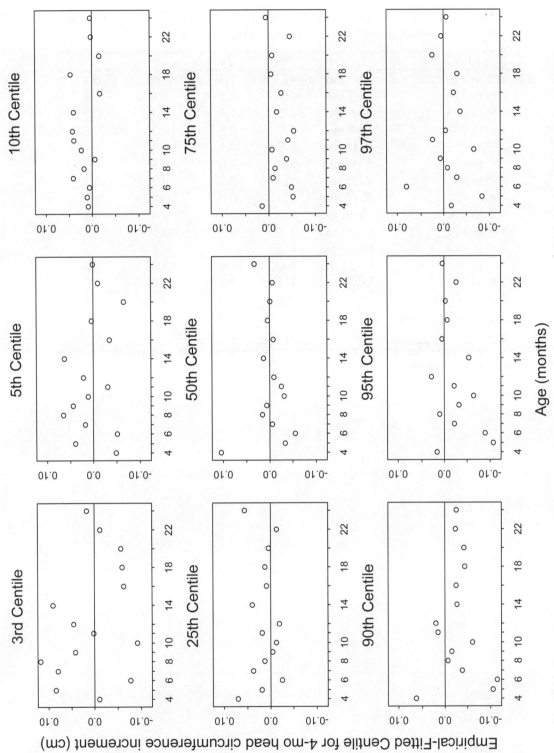

Figure A5.30 Centile residuals from fitting selected model for 4-month head circumference velocity for girls

A5.4a 6-month intervals for boys

Table A5.7   **Q-test for z-scores from selected model [BCPE(x=age$^{0.05}$, df(μ)=9, df(σ)=4, df(ν)=2, τ=2)] for 6-month head circumference velocity for boys**

Age (days)	Group	N	z1	z2	z3
175 to 198	**0-6 mo**	423	1.5	1.5	-0.4
198 to 229	**1-7 mo**	416	-0.5	-0.8	0.8
229 to 259	**2-8 mo**	415	-1.4	-1.1	0.7
259 to 289	**3-9 mo**	407	0.5	-0.7	0.5
289 to 320	**4-10 mo**	402	0.5	0.3	0.8
320 to 350	**5-11 mo**	414	0.0	0.1	-0.2
350 to 396	**6-12 mo**	418	-0.2	-0.3	-0.2
396 to 457	**8-14 mo**	411	0.0	0.0	-1.9
457 to 518	**10-16 mo**	403	-0.2	1.4	0.3
518 to 579	**12-18 mo**	410	0.0	-0.5	-0.3
579 to 640	**14-20 mo**	415	-0.2	0.4	1.3
640 to 701	**16-22 mo**	408	0.0	-0.3	-0.1
701 to 750	**18-24 mo**	410	0.2	0.0	0.6
Overall Q stats		5352	5.3	7.1	8.3
degrees of freedom			4.0	10.5	11.0
p-value			0.2586	0.7562	0.6846

Note: Absolute values of z1, z2 or z3 larger than 2 indicate misfit of, respectively, mean, variance or skewness.

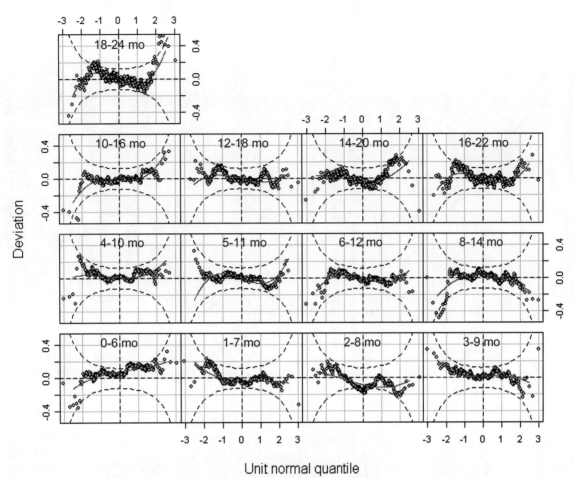

Unit normal quantile

Figure A5.31 Worm plots from selected model [BCPE(x=age$^{0.05}$, df(μ)=9, df(σ)=4, df(ν)=2, τ=2)] for 6-month head circumference velocity for boys

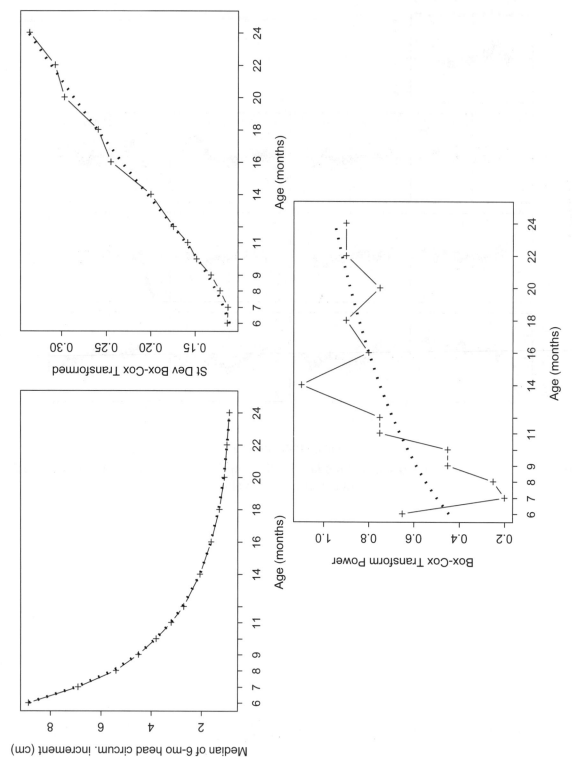

Figure A5.32 Fitting of the μ, σ, and ν curves of selected model for 6-month head circumference velocity for boys

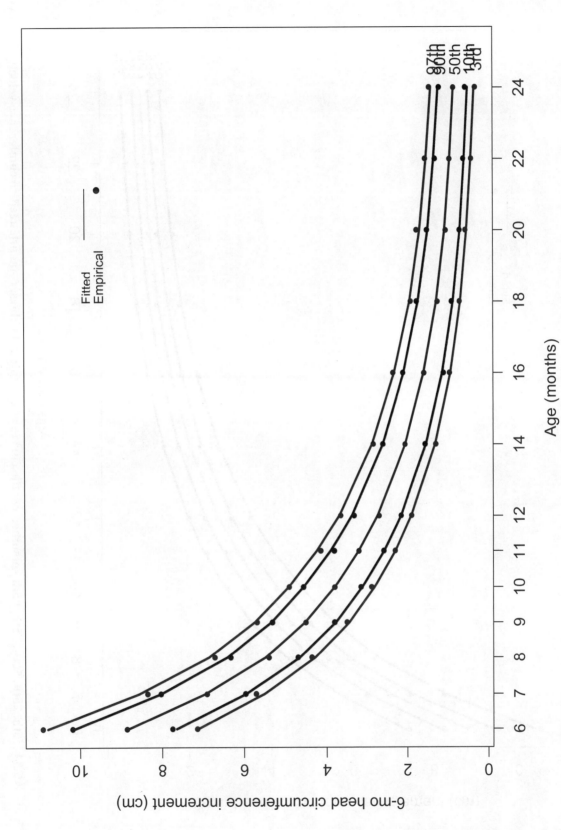

Figure A5.33   3rd, 10th, 50th, 90th, 97th smoothed centile curves and empirical values: 6-month head circumference velocity for boys

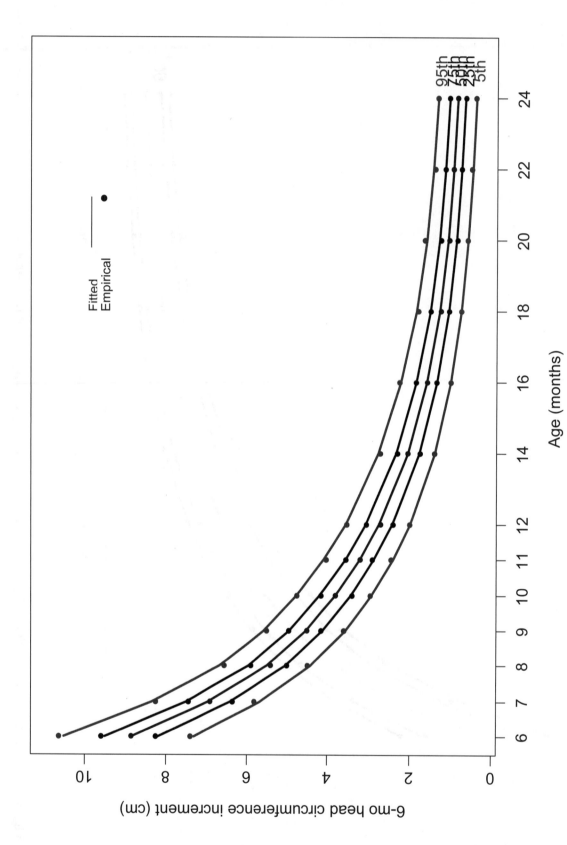

Figure A5.34   5th, 25th, 50th, 75th, 95th smoothed centile curves and empirical values: 6-month head circumference velocity for boys

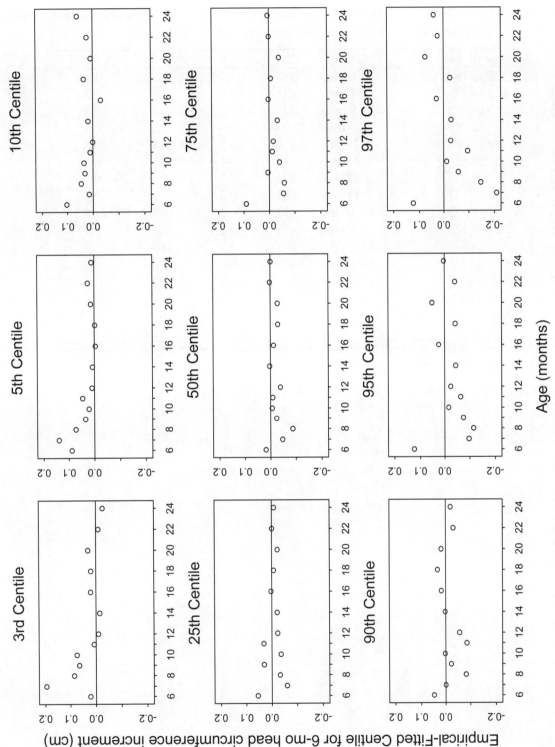

Figure A5.35 Centile residuals from fitting selected model for 6-month head circumference velocity for boys

A5.4b 6-month intervals for girls

Table A5.8   **Q-test for z-scores from selected model [BCPE(x=age$^{0.05}$, df(µ)=9, df(σ)=5, df(v)=2, τ=2)] for 6-month head circumference velocity for girls**

Age (days)	Group	N	z1	z2	z3
178 to 198	**0-6 mo**	447	1.7	0.7	-1.8
198 to 229	**1-7 mo**	443	-0.9	-0.8	1.4
229 to 259	**2-8 mo**	439	-1.2	-0.3	0.9
259 to 289	**3-9 mo**	443	0.5	0.6	-0.8
289 to 320	**4-10 mo**	439	0.2	0.1	0.8
320 to 350	**5-11 mo**	440	0.1	-1.2	0.9
350 to 396	**6-12 mo**	447	0.1	0.5	-0.2
396 to 457	**8-14 mo**	444	-0.3	0.0	0.1
457 to 518	**10-16 mo**	437	0.3	0.1	1.8
518 to 579	**12-18 mo**	448	-0.2	-0.5	-0.9
579 to 640	**14-20 mo**	443	-0.2	0.6	-1.3
640 to 701	**16-22 mo**	432	-0.9	2.6	0.9
701 to 749	**18-24 mo**	444	0.8	-2.0	0.3
Overall Q stats		5746	7.3	15.0	14.7
degrees of freedom			4.0	10.0	11.0
p-value			0.1226	0.1310	0.1967

Note: Absolute values of z1, z2 or z3 larger than 2 indicate misfit of, respectively, mean, variance or skewness.

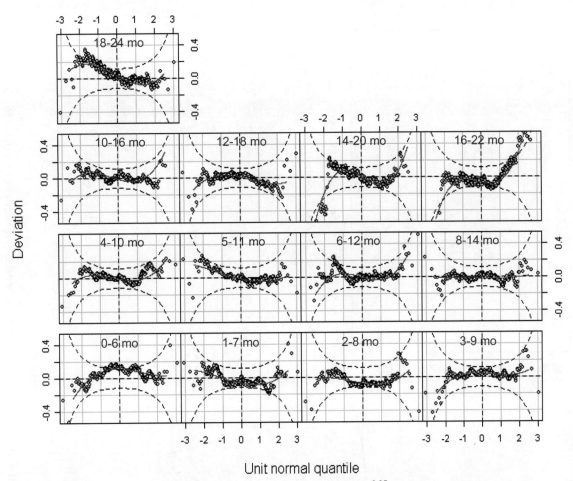

Figure A5.36 Worm plots from selected model [BCPE(x=age$^{0.05}$, df(μ)=9, df(σ)=5, df(ν)=2, τ=2)] for 6-month head circumference velocity for girls

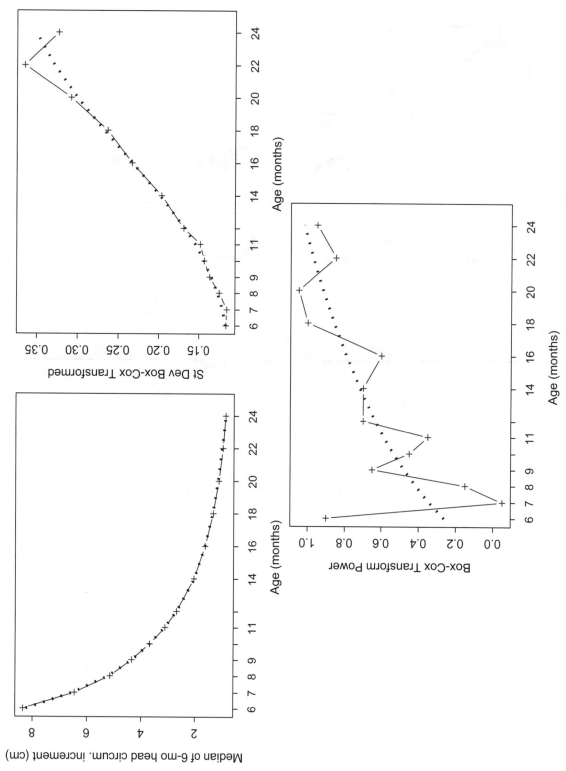

Figure A5.37 Fitting of the μ, σ, and ν curves of selected model for 6-month head circumference velocity for girls

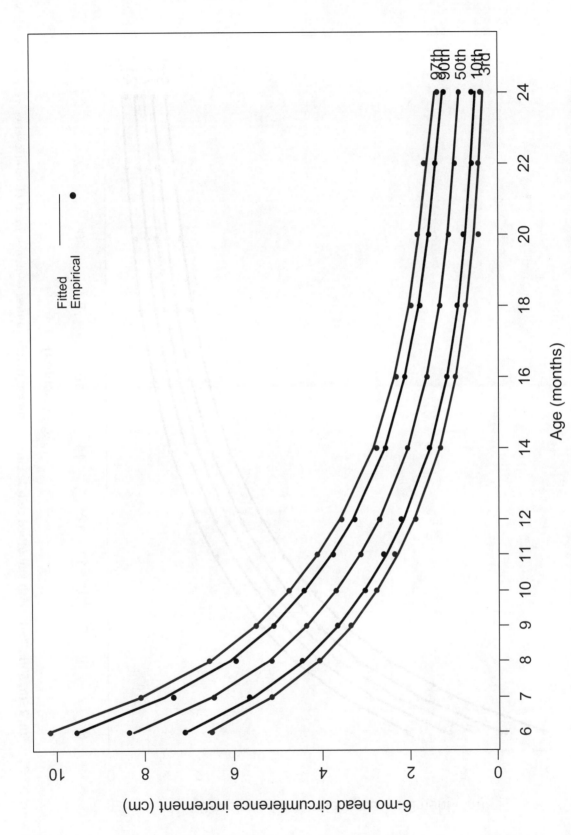

Figure A5.38 3rd, 10th, 50th, 90th, 97th smoothed centile curves and empirical values: 6-month head circumference velocity for girls

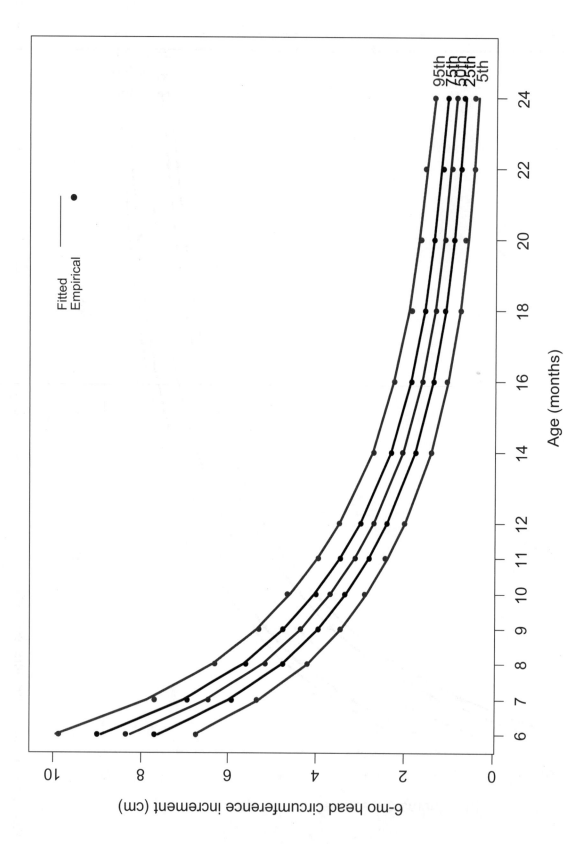

Figure A5.39   5th, 25th, 50th, 75th, 95th smoothed centile curves and empirical values: 6-month head circumference velocity for girls

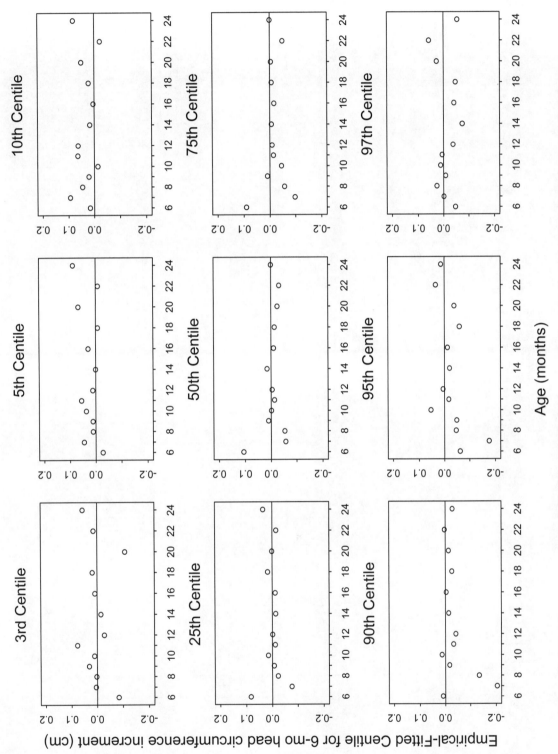

Figure A5.40 Centile residuals from fitting selected model for 6-month head circumference velocity for girls

6. COMPUTATION OF CENTILES AND Z-SCORES FOR VELOCITIES BASED ON WEIGHT, LENGTH AND HEAD CIRCUMFERENCE

The same method used to calculate centiles and z-scores for the attained growth standards based on weight is used to calculate centiles and z-scores for the velocity standards based on weight, length and head circumference increments. Briefly, the computation of percentiles and z-scores for these standards uses formulae based on a restricted application of the LMS method as used for the attained growth weight-based indicators, limiting the Box-Cox normal distribution to the interval corresponding to z-scores where empirical data were available (i.e. between -3 SD and +3 SD). Beyond these limits, the standard deviation at each age was fixed to the distance between ±2 SD and ±3 SD, respectively. This approach avoids making assumptions about the distribution of data beyond the limits of the observed values (WHO Multicentre Growth Reference Study Group, 2006a).

Adjustment to the basic methodology had to be applied for weight velocities conditional on age (see section 2.5). Children experience weight losses and, consequently, weight increments occur in negative values while the BCPE distribution can handle only positive values. Thus, before the BCPE could be applied to these data, it was necessary to add a constant value δ (delta) to all increments to shift their distribution above zero and, subsequently, to subtract delta from the predicted centiles. To calculate individual z scores, δ is first added to the child's increment and then the L, M and S values of the model are fitted on the shifted observations. When a child's increment is less than -δ (i.e. the increment is negative and its absolute value is greater than δ), the correction applied for skewed attained growth standards beyond -3 SD or +3 SD will be used, since in reality such an increment lies below -3 SD.

For all indicators, the tabulated fitted values of Box-Cox power, median and coefficient of variation corresponding to the visit age t are denoted by $L(t)$, $M(t)$ and $S(t)$, respectively.

Centiles and z-scores for weight velocities conditional on age

Note that in this case, the values of $L(t)$, $M(t)$ and $S(t)$ are based on the shifted BCPE distribution. Given the value of δ for the corresponding standard, the centiles were calculated as follows:

$$C_{100\alpha}(t) = M(t)\left[1 + L(t)S(t)Z_\alpha\right]^{1/L(t)} - \delta, \qquad -3 \le Z_\alpha \le 3$$

The following procedure is recommended to calculate a z-score for an individual child with weight increment y at the visit age t:

1. Calculate

$$z_{ind} = \frac{\left[\dfrac{(y+\delta)}{M(t)}\right]^{L(t)} - 1}{S(t)L(t)}$$

2. Compute the final z-score $\left(z_{ind}^*\right)$ of the child for that indicator as:

$$z_{ind}^* = \begin{cases} z_{ind} & if \quad |z_{ind}| \le 3 \\[2mm] 3 + \left(\dfrac{(y+\delta)-SD3pos}{SD23pos}\right) & if \quad z_{ind} > 3 \\[2mm] -3 + \left(\dfrac{(y+\delta)-SD3neg}{SD23neg}\right) & if \quad z_{ind} < -3 \end{cases}$$

where

$SD3pos$ is the cut-off +3 SD calculated at t by the LMS method:

$$SD3pos = M(t)[1 + L(t)*S(t)*(3)]^{1/L(t)};$$

$SD3neg$ is the cut-off -3 SD calculated at t by the LMS method:

$$SD3neg = M(t)[1 + L(t)*S(t)*(-3)]^{1/L(t)};$$

$SD23pos$ is the difference between the cut-offs +3 SD and +2 SD calculated at t by the LMS method:

$$SD23pos = M(t)[1 + L(t)*S(t)*(3)]^{1/L(t)} - M(t)[1 + L(t)*S(t)*(2)]^{1/L(t)};$$

and $SD23neg$ is the difference between the cut-offs -2 SD and -3 SD calculated at t by the LMS method:

$$SD23neg = M(t)[1 + L(t)*S(t)*(-2)]^{1/L(t)} - M(t)[1 + L(t)*S(t)*(-3)]^{1/L(t)}$$

To illustrate the procedure, examples with the 2-month interval weight velocity conditional on age for boys follow.

Child 1: 6-month-old boy with an increment, i.e. weight gain 2200 g between 4 and 6 months.

L=0.5891;   M=1541.3670;   S=0.20130;   δ=600;

$$z_{ind} = \frac{\left[\dfrac{(2200+600)}{1541.3670}\right]^{0.5891} - 1}{0.20130*0.5891} = 3.55 \quad \textbf{>3}$$

$$SD3pos = 1541.3670 * \left[1 + (0.5891) * 0.20130 * (3)\right]^{1/(0.5891)} = 2583.96$$

$$SD2pos = 1541.3670 * \left[1 + (0.5891) * 0.20130 * (2)\right]^{1/(0.5891)} = 2212.11$$

$$SD23pos = 2583.96 - 2212.11 = 371.85$$

$$\Rightarrow z_{ind}^* = 3 + \left(\frac{(2200 + 600) - 2583.96}{371.85}\right) = 3.58$$

Child 2: 18-month-old boy with an increment of -500 g (weight loss of 500 g) between 16 and 18 months.

L=0.8078;   M=1000.9680;   S=0.31615;   δ=600;

$$z_{ind} = \frac{\left[\left.(-500 + 600)\right/1000.9680\right]^{0.8078} - 1}{0.31615 * 0.8078} = -3.31 \quad \text{<-3}$$

$$SD2neg = 1000.9680 * \left[1 + 0.8078 * 0.31615 * (-2)\right]^{1/0.8078} = 413.10$$

$$SD3neg = 1000.9680 * \left[1 + 0.8078 * 0.31615 * (-3)\right]^{1/0.8078} = 165.65$$

$$SD23neg = 413.10 - 165.65 = 247.45$$

$$\Rightarrow z_{ind}^* = -3 + \left(\frac{(-500 + 600) - 165.65}{247.45}\right) = -3.27$$

Child 3: 13-month-old boy with a weight gain of 1200 g between 11 and 13 months.

L=0.7191;   M=1057.9071;   S=0.28462;   δ=600;

$$z_{ind} = \frac{\left[\left.(1200 + 600)\right/1057.9071\right]^{0.7191} - 1}{0.0.7191 * 0.28462} = 2.27 \quad \text{≥-3 and ≤3}\quad \textbf{(LMS z-score)}$$

Centiles and z-scores for length and head circumference velocities conditional on age

The centiles were calculated as follows:

$$C_{100\alpha}(t) = M(t)\left[1 + L(t)S(t)Z_\alpha\right]^{1/L(t)}, \quad -3 \leq Z_\alpha \leq 3$$

The following procedure is recommended to calculate a z-score for an individual child with length or head circumference increment y at the visit age t:

1. Calculate

$$z_{ind} = \frac{\left[y/M(t)\right]^{L(t)} - 1}{S(t)L(t)}$$

2. Compute the final z-score $\left(z_{ind}^*\right)$ of the child for that indicator as:

$$z_{ind}^* = \begin{cases} z_{ind} & if \quad \left|z_{ind}\right| \leq 3 \\[2ex] 3 + \left(\dfrac{y - SD3pos}{SD23pos}\right) & if \quad z_{ind} > 3 \\[2ex] -3 + \left(\dfrac{y - SD3neg}{SD23neg}\right) & if \quad z_{ind} < -3 \end{cases}$$

where

$SD3pos$ is the cut-off +3 SD calculated at t by the LMS method:

$$SD3pos = M(t)\left[1 + L(t) * S(t) * (3)\right]^{1/L(t)};$$

$SD3neg$ is the cut-off -3 SD calculated at t by the LMS method:

$$SD3neg = M(t)\left[1 + L(t) * S(t) * (-3)\right]^{1/L(t)};$$

$SD23pos$ is the difference between the cut-offs +3 SD and +2 SD calculated at t by the LMS method:

$$SD23pos = M(t)\left[1 + L(t) * S(t) * (3)\right]^{1/L(t)} - M(t)\left[1 + L(t) * S(t) * (2)\right]^{1/L(t)};$$

and *SD23neg* is the difference between the cut-offs -2 SD and -3 SD calculated at *t* by the LMS method:

$$SD23neg = M(t)[1 + L(t)*S(t)*(-2)]^{1/L(t)} - M(t)[1 + L(t)*S(t)*(-3)]^{1/L(t)}$$

To illustrate the procedure, examples with the 3-month interval length velocity conditional on age for girls follow.

Child 1: 12-month-old girl with an increment, i.e. length gain 7.5 cm between 9 and 12 months.

L=0.8538;   M=3.8692;   S=0.23503;

$$z_{ind} = \frac{\left[7.5 \big/ 3.8692 \right]^{0.8538} - 1}{0.23503*0.8538} = 3.79 \quad \mathbf{>3}$$

$$SD3pos = 3.8692*[1 + 0.8538*0.23503*(3)]^{1/0.8538} = 6.72$$
$$SD2pos = 3.8692*[1 + 0.8538*0.23503*(2)]^{1/0.8538} = 5.74$$
$$SD23pos = 6.72 - 5.74 = 0.98$$
$$\Rightarrow \quad z^*_{ind} = 3 + \left(\frac{7.5 - 6.72}{0.98} \right) = 3.80$$

Child 2: 18-month-old girl with an increment of 0.5 cm between 15 and 18 months.

L=0.8538;   M=3.2051;   S=0.28388;

$$z_{ind} = \frac{\left[0.5 \big/ 3.2051 \right]^{0.8538} - 1}{0.28388*0.8538} = -3.28 \quad \mathbf{<-3}$$

$$SD2neg = 3.2051*[1 + 0.8538*0.28388*(-2)]^{1/0.8538} = 1.47$$
$$SD3neg = 3.2051*[1 + 0.8538*0.28388*(-3)]^{1/0.8538} = 0.70$$
$$SD23neg = 1.47 - 0.70 = 0.77$$
$$\Rightarrow \quad z^*_{ind} = -3 + \left(\frac{0.5 - 0.70}{0.77} \right) = -3.26$$

Child 3: 6-month-old girl with a length gain of 8.0 cm between 3 and 6 months.

L=0.8538;   M=5.9428;   S=0.17798;

$$z_{ind} = \frac{\left[8.0 \big/ 5.9428 \right]^{0.8538} - 1}{0.17798*0.8538} = 1.90 \quad \mathbf{\geq -3 \text{ and } \leq 3} \quad \textbf{(LMS z-score)}$$

7. DISCUSSION

The intrinsic biological complexity of the dynamics of human growth made the construction of the standards presented in this report more challenging than was the case for the attained growth standards (WHO Multicentre Growth Reference Study Group, 2006a; 2007). This section seeks to provide guidance for the use and interpretation of the standards based on insights gained during construction of the velocity standards and feedback from clinicians who participated in reviewing and field-testing the velocity tools.

The standards are presented for the age span birth to 24 months. They include weight, length and head circumference centiles conditional on age, in variable measurement intervals. Additionally for weight, empirical centiles of velocity in 1- or 2-week intervals from birth to 60 days are presented. With the exception of tables 15 and 17 (velocity in g/d), all velocity tools of the WHO Child Growth Standards are increment standards describing the distribution of growth increments over variable intervals. As is the case for attained growth, the standards presented in this report are sex-specific. Appendix B summarizes specifications of the BCPE models for each of the growth velocity standards.

Velocity conditional on age

The overall pattern of the (age-conditioned) centiles depicts the age-dependent changes in velocity that characterize human postnatal growth. Growth progresses at a rapidly decelerating rate from birth, reaching a near-plateau by the end of the first year and continues to taper off gently through the second year. This is the expected overall pattern of growth under conditions of adequate nutrition and psychosocial care with no chronic infections or unusual rates and/or severity of acute infections: the pattern that underpins the general expectation that infants will double their weight by age 6 months and triple it by 12 months. However, examination of individual growth trajectories has shown saltatory increments in short ($\leq$24 hours) intervals followed by periods (2-63 days) of no measurable growth (Lampl et al., 1992). Although the intervals (1- to 6-months) presented for the main age-conditioned tools of these standards cannot capture the short-span saltation and stasis described by Lampl and co-workers, the growth velocities of individual children in the WHO standards are characterized by very high variability in consecutive growth intervals. It is not unusual for a child to grow at the 95th velocity centile one month and at the 20th the next while continuing to track on the attained weight-for-age chart. Alternating or irregular patterns of high and low velocities may occur in successive periods even in the absence of morbidity. With regard to weight, losses or slow gains (related to morbidity or otherwise) in a given period are normally followed by higher velocities, likely indicating catch-up growth.

The 1-, 2-, 3-, 4- and 6-month increment tables are independent of each other and the clinician should use the one that most closely approximates the interval over which the child is seen. For example, the centile corresponding to an increment between age 2 and 3 months is not associated with the centile corresponding to half of the increment in the 2-month interval between ages 1 and 3 months. This is because one cannot expect the growth rate in a given 2-month period, except perhaps at the median, to be the sum of the two corresponding 1-month intervals.

With specific reference to weight, negative increments occur generally after 6 months of age and are captured in the lowest centiles. They coincide with the weaning period, when children are more exposed to food contamination, and when they become more active and start to explore their environment. Others who have developed velocity references have observed similar losses (WHO Working Group on Infant Growth, 1994), even if final published figures did not include them since only a narrow range of centiles were presented (Guo et al., 1991; Roche et al., 1989). It is important to note that losses that are tolerable in short intervals might not be acceptable in longer intervals. For example, the 5th centile indicates a loss of about 100g between 10 and 11 months and also between 11 and 12 months (Table 4), which can be acceptable for 1-month intervals at that age. However, the same 5th centile for a 2-month interval at the same age (10 to 12 months) indicates a gain of about 30g (Table 6), implying that there was time for recovery within the longer interval.

Alternative approaches to constructing conditional weight gain references

Others have approached the construction of conditional weight gain references by applying methodologies that adjust not only for age but also for regression to the mean (Wright et al, 1994; Cole, 1995; Cole, 1997). The theoretical basis for this approach is the expectation that over time infant weights drift towards the median from the tails of the distribution. Using this approach, weight gain is calculated in terms of the change (compared with the initial measurement) in the infant's attained weight SD score adjusted for regression to the mean (Cole, 1995). The formula for this calculation hinges on the correlation between the initial and second SD scores, which determines the expected slope of the change in the child's size between the two points of measurement. Despite its theoretical advantages, calculation of this conditional gain SD score requires computerization and thus limits the potential for its application. In effect, this approach has not gained currency in clinical settings.

To explore how conditional gain SD scores compare with the increment centiles presented in this report, the published methodology (Cole, 1995) was applied for adjusting for regression to the mean on 1- and 2-month interval weight increments (results are presented in Appendix C). The first step was to calculate the attained weight-for-age (WA) z-score for each child at each of the visits. Next, the respective correlation matrices for the 1- and 2-month intervals were derived. Then, the published formula to calculate SD_{gain} (the z-score associated with the change in WA z-score between visits) was applied. The SD_{gain} values were compared with z-scores of the age-conditioned 1- and 2-month weight increments.

Plots of empirical densities showed that the distributions of the z-scores from the two methods overlap for each respective test interval (figures C1 and C2). Distributions of pairwise differences between the z-scores from the two methods were also examined (figures C3 and C4). Ninety percent of the differences were between -0.33 and +0.34 (for 1-month intervals) and between -0.27 and +0.29 (for 2-month intervals).

To assess the magnitude of the impact of regression to the mean, two sets of children were selected: one in the lower bound (WA z-scores between -2.5 and -1.5) and the other in the upper bound (WA z-scores between +1.5 to +2.5) of attained growth at the start (time1) of specified intervals. The change in their z-scores at the end (time2) of 1- or 2-month periods were examined to observe what proportion deviated from the assumption of regression to the mean (Table C1).

For the lower bound (time1 z-scores between -2.5 and -1.5), the results were consistent with regression to the mean only for initial ages 0-1 months and 0-2 months, i.e. WA drifted further from the median for 21% and 13% of children, respectively. For the remaining ages, 30-52% (1-month intervals) and 28-47% (2-month intervals) of weights shifted further from the mean, contrary to shifts that would have reflected regression to the mean. Similar findings were observed for the upper bound (time1 z-scores between +1.5 and +2.5) i.e. 27% (age 0-1 month) and 20% (age 0-2 months) drifted away from the mean. In the older age groups, this tendency was observed for 37-55% (1-month intervals) and 30-54% (2-month intervals). As expected, corresponding average changes in WA z-scores were, relatively high at ages 0-1 or 0-2 months (in the assumed direction of regression to the mean), but they dropped rapidly thereafter to near 0.

In summary, growth in snapshots of 1- or 2-month intervals was consistent with regression to the mean between birth and 1 or 2 months but the phenomenon was much less evident at later ages. Differences between individual z-scores when applying the two methods were relatively minor. This raises questions regarding the impact those differences have on clinical management and the method's conceptual and practical accessibility for users in disparate settings. For the age period when the largest impact of regression to the mean is observed, as described below this report provides sex-specific centiles for weight increments conditional on birth weight in 1- and 2-week intervals from birth to 2 months.

Tables of weight velocity from birth to 60 days

These tables present physiological weight losses that occur in the early postnatal period but that are not usually included in available reference data.

In-depth comparisons between the sexes were made in the process of deriving these centiles. In most cases, boys' net increments in the 2-week intervals between 14 and 60 days were higher than girls' increments by values of 50-100 g. The differences in the first two weeks (birth to 7 and 7-14 days) were less clear-cut, but it was interesting to observe that the weight losses (depicted in the 5th and 10th centiles) between birth and day 7 were slightly attenuated in girls compared to boys.

It was not possible to estimate from these data precisely when infants should recover their birth weight following weight loss that is common in the first few postnatal days. Net increments at the median (0 to 7 days) are positive for both boys and girls, suggesting that recovery of birth weight could be achieved in less than one week. Considering the 25th centile (0 g increment from birth to 7 days), the data suggest that 75% of newborns recover their birth weight by day 7. It is understood that recovery depends on what percentage of birth weight was lost and successful initiation of lactation. However, rather than focus only on weight gain, it is important to adopt a holistic approach by looking at the child's overall health status and clinical signs. This involves also assessing mother-child interaction, indicators of successful breastfeeding such as infant breastfeeding behaviour and the timing of stage II lactogenesis (i.e. the onset of a copious milk supply), and breastfeeding technique (position and attachment), as these are necessary for maintaining successful infant nutrition. The overall breastfeeding profile and some aspects of its initiation among the infants included in these standards were published elsewhere (WHO Multicentre Growth Reference Study Group, 2006d).

The complexity of growth velocity is not adequately reflected in the usual presentation of gross estimations of growth rate over wide age spans. Such estimations overlook the dramatic changes that characterize growth in the first few months and the high variability within an individual child's growth rate in succeeding intervals. These centiles (birth to 60 days) provide a description of weekly and biweekly changes in velocity, illustrating the inadequacy of rules of thumb such as "infants should gain 200 g/week or 30 g/d in the first 3 months".

Centiles are presented both for net increments and for velocity in g/d. It is important to note that the g/d figures are not the simple average of the gross gains or losses reported in corresponding weekly and fortnightly tables. The g/d figures are derived by calculating individual daily increments for newborns in each of the birth weight categories and then estimating centiles directly from the raw g/d values. When mother-child dyads experience breastfeeding difficulties in the early postpartum period, lactation performance and weight gain are monitored every few days, hence increments per day are likely to be handier to use than weekly or fortnightly increments. Even in the absence of such difficulties, visits to the clinic take place at random ages, and these daily increments offer a flexible option for evaluating growth over fractions of the tabulated time blocks. It is important to note that the g/d figures, particularly in the first week, are composite figures reflecting, on average, losses followed by recovery.

Contrary to speculation that weight velocity would vary by birth weight, the centiles from the various birth-weight categories were very similar, leading to the conclusion that velocities can be collapsed into a single column. Low or high anthropometric values observed in the WHO standards represent the physiological extremes of normality among children in the absence of intrauterine growth problems. If this were not the case, a negative correlation between birth weight and early growth rate would have been more likely because postnatal catch-up and catch-down growth would have been observed.

Minimum weight gain tables

Tables of weight gain conditional on starting weight were requested by users of the table of "expected minimum gains in weight" in community-based growth promotion programmes mainly in Central America (Griffiths et al., 1996; Griffiths and McGuire, 2005). The AIN (*Atención Integral al Niño*) tables were developed using data from 112 children born between 1972 and 1974 and followed from birth to 2 years by the *Centro Latinoamericano de Perinatología* (Martell et al., 1981). The values of expected weight do not take into account sex or age, and it appears that the weight gain selected as the minimum was the 25th centile; otherwise, little is known about them (Martorell et al., 2002). The original AIN table provides single values of expected minimum weight gains in 30-day or 60-day intervals relative to the child's starting weight.

Tables of 1- and 2-month weight gains conditional on starting weight were produced and circulated for peer review. Reviewers rejected them on substantive grounds, and they were thus excluded from the final standards.

Firstly, the basic assumption of the AIN table, i.e. that young children of the same weight grow at the same rate irrespective of age, is flawed. In the WHO standards, starting at 5 kg, there is a significant negative association between age and final weight. This implies that younger children at the same starting weight end up with a higher final weight after 1- and 2-month intervals compared to those at older ages.

Secondly, it is impossible to select "expected minimum weight gains" that would be appropriate for all infants or children with the same starting weight. Such values are bound to be too low for some infants/children and too high for others of the same starting weight. Moreover, the selection of single minimum thresholds introduces the notion of centile tracking in velocity that is contrary to normal physiological growth in individual children. In the WHO standards, the probability of two consecutive 1-month or 2-month weight increments falling below the 5th centile is 0.3%. If the 15th centile is chosen, this probability increases to only 2% and 1.8%, respectively.

Thirdly, as infants grow older the lower centile values (25th and below) become less than the day-to-day variability in weight, making detection of a minimum weight at this level impossible. Examining the 1-month interval centiles for boys, for starting weights greater than about 8.5 kg, the 25th centile value for final weight is only 100 g greater than the starting weight. The day-to-day variability (SD) is about twice this level. For girls, 100 g differences are seen between starting and 25th centile final weights at even lower weights, e.g. about 8 kg. For girls that start at 12.7 kg, the 25th centile final weight is 100 g less than the starting weight. The situation is even worse if the 15th or 5th centiles are selected (e.g. examining the 1-month interval for girls, a starting weight of 12 kg implies a loss of 100 g and 200 g in the final weight for the 15th and 5th centile, respectively).

Overall considerations

Measurement error. Measurements of growth are subject to error from multiple sources. Faulty measurements can lead to grossly erroneous judgements regarding a child's growth. The accuracy of growth assessment is improved greatly if measurements are replicated independently and the values averaged. This procedure minimizes the impact of faulty single measurements. MGRS measurements were undertaken to assure the highest level of reliability; and the final values used in the creation of these standards were an average of two observations, thereby minimizing random measurement errors in observed growth. This level of reliability is not typical in routine clinical measurement in primary health care settings; however, it can be achieved in research contexts (WHO Multicentre Growth Reference Study Group, 2006b) and where resources permit, in clinical situations caring for children at high risk of growth problems. The training course on child growth assessment is a tool to assist health care providers in the effective application of the WHO growth standards. It teaches, inter alia, the knowledge and skills needed to measure children correctly (WHO, 2008).

Measurement intervals in field application. Ideally, velocity assessment should be done at scheduled visits that coincide with the ages and intervals (1, 2, 3, 4 or 6 months) for which the centiles are presented. In practice, however, the timing of clinic visits is dictated by uncontrollable factors, and ingenuity will be called for in applying the standards. In constructing the standards, some variation was allowed around the intervals. For measurements made at ages 0-6 months, 6-12 months and 12-24 months, the allowable deviations from the exact planned age were ±3 days, ±5 days and ±7 days, respectively. The practical advantage of this approach is that use of the standards allows for equally slight deviations without a need to correct observed increments through interpolation. For example, to assess a two-month increment between 11 months and 13 months of age the observed increment could be validly used as long as the first measurement was no more than 5 days early or late and the second measurement no more than 7 days early or late.

The simplest approach to dealing with measurement intervals beyond allowable ranges is to interpolate (i.e. prorate) observed increments to the relevant interval or to refer to the next larger interval if appropriate. For example, a boy weighed at 11 months returns at 13 months and 24 days having gained 600 g. If this increment is prorated to the 2-month interval 11-13 months, the estimated gain is 429 g (600 g/84 days × 60 days), which is just below the 50th centile (458 g, Table 6). If the 3-month interval 11-14 months is referred to instead, there is no need to interpolate as the visit falls within the allowable difference (±7 days); his increment (600 g) also is just below the 50th centile (665 g, Table 8). The assumption made is that the rate of growth was constant over this period, but there is no alternative way of partitioning the increment.

If the observed interval is on target, say exactly 2 months, but the starting and ending ages do not coincide with those tabulated in the standards (e.g. an increment measured over the exact 2-month interval between 11.4 and 13.4 months of age), the recommended practical solution is to use the tabulated reference values for the 11 to 13-month age interval. Similarly, for an increment observed between 11.6 and 13.6 months of age one would use the reference values tabulated for the 12 to 14-month interval. It should be understood that these are compromises whose limitations are especially apparent in the first year when growth decelerates rapidly and the difference in velocity between consecutive periods can be large. For example, growth between 2.5 to 3.5 months carries equal contributions from 2-3 and 3-4 month intervals: a baby girl who gained 310 g would be classified as below the 3rd centile at 2-3 months and as below the 15th centile at 3-4 months. The best clinical judgement in such circumstances requires making a holistic assessment of the child's health. A more precise option in the forgoing case (i.e. when interval length is on target) is to interpolate the L, M and S values from consecutive age intervals and to calculate the child's z-score as described in Chapter 6.

Clinical usefulness of growth velocity. The questions that a clinician seeks to answer when using a velocity standard include whether a child's growth rate over a specified interval, or over a series of intervals, raises concern about underlying morbidity; or in the context of interventions to promote growth (e.g. in endocrinology), whether a given treatment produced the expected change in growth rate; or, for the newborn, if breastfeeding has been successfully established.

There are some fundamental differences between velocity and attained (distance) growth that affect how the increment standards should be used and interpreted. Chief among them is the lack of correlation between successive increments in healthy, normally growing children. For individual attained growth curves, the variability in successive z-scores tends to be minimal over short periods (there are high correlations between successive attained values). This "tracking" is not usually seen for successive individual growth velocities. For example, as indicated earlier, the probability of two consecutive 1-month or 2-month weight increments falling below the 5th centile is 0.3%. If the 15th centile is chosen, this probability increases to only 2% and 1.8%, respectively. Normally growing children can have a very high z-score one month and a very low one the following month, or vice versa, without any underlying reason for concern. Thus, a single low value is uninformative; only when velocities are repeatedly low should they cause concern. Nevertheless, very low z-score values, even if observed only once, should raise the question of whether there is underlying morbidity within the holistic clinical assessment of the child.

Some authors recommend that two successive increments below a cut-off like the 5th centile be used (Roche and Sun, 2003). Others suggest that consecutive increments below the 25th centile should signal growth problems (Healy et al., 1988). Healy and co-workers chose this limit on the basis that the chance of a false positive diagnosis (i.e. a normally growing child with two successive increments below this centile) is approximately 6.25% (0.25^2). This raises an important question: Does the interval matter, for example, if these low velocities occur in two consecutive 1-month versus 3-month intervals? We think it does when we consider the cumulative effect of growth deficits. Future research will need to determine what patterns of successive velocity thresholds over which specified intervals have the best diagnostic and prognostic validity for specific diseases. The need for this type of clinical research applies to both high and low velocities.

During periods of severe illness (e.g. prolonged diarrhoea), one would expect very low velocity followed by compensatory high velocity (catch-up). During catch-up growth, one would expect successive increments to be repeatedly in the higher ranges. An important difference with attained growth is that single extreme values of increments are comparatively less worrisome. For example, z-scores above +6 and below -6 for attained growth are observed only in very rare conditions like severe dwarfism, gigantism, severe cachexia and extreme obesity. However, such extreme z-score values may be seen during the assessment of growth velocity. Ultimately, growth velocity must always be interpreted in conjunction with attained growth, as the position on the attained growth chart is essential to interpreting the growth rate, e.g., low weight velocity if the child is overweight and catching down, or higher weight velocity reflecting catch-up growth when recovering from illness.

8. BIBLIOGRAPHY

Baumgartner RN, Roche AF, Himes JH (1986). Incremental growth tables. *American Journal of Clinical Nutrition*, 43:711–22.

Bhandari N, Bahl R, Taneja S, de Onis M, Bhan MK (2002). Growth performance of affluent Indian children is similar to that in developed countries. *Bulletin of the World Health Organization*, 80:189–195.

Borghi E, de Onis M, Garza C, van den Broeck J, Frongillo EA, Grummer-Strawn L, van Buuren S, Pan H, Molinari L, Martorell R, Onyango AW, Martines JC for the WHO Multicentre Growth Reference Study Group (2006). Construction of the World Health Organization child growth standards: selection of methods for attained growth curves. *Statistics in Medicine*, 25:247–265.

Cole TJ, Green PJ (1992). Smoothing reference centile curves: the LMS method and penalized likelihood. *Statistics in Medicine*, 11:1305–1319.

Cole TJ (1995). Conditional reference charts to assess weight gain in British infants. *Archives of Disease in Childhood*, 73:8–16.

Cole TJ (1997). 3-in-1 weight monitoring chart [research letter]. *Lancet*, 349:102–103.

Cole TJ (1998). Presenting information on growth distance and conditional velocity in one chart: practical issues of chart design. *Statistics in Medicine*, 17:2697–2707.

de Onis M, Garza C, Victora CG, Bhan MK, Norum KR, eds. (2004a). WHO Multicentre Growth Reference Study (MGRS): Rationale, planning and implementation. *Food and Nutrition Bulletin*, 25(Suppl. 1):S1–S89.

de Onis M, Garza C, Victora CG, Onyango AW, Frongillo EA, Martines J, for the WHO Multicentre Growth Reference Study Group (2004b). The WHO Multicentre Growth Reference Study: planning, study design and methodology. *Food and Nutrition Bulletin*, 25(Suppl. 1):S15–S26.

de Onis M, Onyango AW, van den Broeck J, Chumlea WC, Martorell R, for the WHO Multicentre Growth Reference Study Group (2004c). Measurement and standardization protocols for anthropometry used in the construction of a new international growth reference. *Food and Nutrition Bulletin*, 25(Suppl. 1):S27–S36.

DiCiccio TJ, Monti, AC (2004). Inferential aspects of the Skew Exponential Power Distribution. *Journal of the American Statistical Association*, 99:439–450.

Falkner F (1958). Some physical measurements in the first three years of life. *Archives of Disease in Childhood*, 33:1–9.

Goldstein H (1986). Efficient statistical modelling of longitudinal data. *Annals of Human Biology*, 13:129–141.

Griffiths M, Dickin K, Favin M (1996). Promoting the Growth of Children: What Works. Rationale and Guidance for Programs. Tool #4, The World Bank Nutrition Toolkit, Washington DC: The World Bank.

Griffiths M, McGuire JS (2005). A New Dimension for Health Reform: The Integrated Community Child Health Program in Honduras. In *Health System Innovations in Central America: Lessons and Impact of New Approaches,* ed. Gerard La Forgia. Washington, DC: World Bank Working Paper 57.

Guo S, Roche AF, Fomon SJ, Nelson SE, Chumlea WC, Rogers RR, Baumgartner RN, Ziegler EE, Siervogel RM (1991). Reference data on gains in weight and length during the first two years of life. *Journal of Pediatrics*, 119:355–62.

Healy MJR, Yang M, Tanner J, Zumrawi Y (1988). The use of short-term increments in length to monitor growth in infancy. In: Waterlow JC, ed. Linear Growth Retardation in Less Developed Countries. Nestlé Nutrition Workshop Series Vol. 14. New York, Vevey/Raven Press.

Himes JH (1999). Minimum time intervals for serial measurements of growth in recumbent length or stature of individual children. *Acta Paediatrica*, 88:120–5.

Himes JH, Frongillo EA (2007). Development of the WHO standards for growth velocity from birth to two years of age: Statistical and technical issues. *Ad hoc Advisory Group meeting on the construction of growth velocity standards*. Geneva, 19-21 March 2007. Background document No. 2.

Jones MC, Pewsey A (2008) Sinh-arcsinh distributions: a broad family giving rise to powerful tests of normality and symmetry. Technical Report 08/06, Statistics Group, The Open University.

Lampl M, Velhuis JD, Johnson ML (1992). Saltation and stasis: A model of human growth. *Science,* 258:801–3.

Martell M, Bertolini LA, Nieto F, Tenzer SM, Ruggia R, and Belitzky R (1981). Crecimiento y desarrollo en los dos primeros años de vida postnatal [Growth and development in the first two years of postanal life]. Washington, DC: Organización Panamericana de la Salud, Publicación Científica N° 406.

Martorell R, Flores R, Hurtado E (2002). Defining growth failure in growth monitoring and promotion programs: comparison of minimum expected weight gain vs. tendency methods. *Summary of a presentation given to the Guatemalan Ministry of Health and to USAID personnel on December 4, 2002.*

Mohamed AJ, Onyango AW, de Onis M, Prakash N, Mabry RM, Alasfoor DH (2004). Socioeconomic predictors of unconstrained child growth in Muscat, Oman. *Eastern Mediterranean Health Journal*, 10:295–302.

Owusu WB, Lartey A, de Onis M, Onyango AW, Frongillo EA (2004). Factors associated with unconstrained growth among affluent Ghanaian children. *Acta Paediatrica*, 93:1115–1119.

Prader A, Largo RH, Molinari L, Issler C (1989). Physical growth of Swiss children from birth to 20 years of age. First Zurich longitudinal study of growth and development. *Helvetica Paediatrica Acta*, 52(Suppl. Jun):1–125.

Roche AF, Himes JH (1980). Incremental growth charts. *American Journal of Clinical Nutrition*, 33(9):2041–2052.

Roche AF, Guo S, Moore WM (1989). Weight and recumbent length from 1 to 12 mo of age: reference data for 1-mo increments. *American Journal of Clinical Nutrition*, 49(4):599–607.

Roche AF, Sun SS (2003). Human growth: assessment and interpretation. Cambridge: Cambridge University Press.

Rigby RA, Stasinopoulos DM (2004). Smooth centile curves for skew and kurtotic data modelled using the Box-Cox power exponential distribution. *Statistics in Medicine*, 23:3053–3076.

Rigby RA, Stasinopoulos DM (2005). Generalized additive models for location, scale and shape. *Journal of the Royal Statistical Society - Series C - Applied Statistics*, 54:507–544.

Royston P, Wright EM (2000). Goodness-of-fit statistics for age-specific reference intervals. *Statistics in Medicine*, 19:2943–2962.

Stasinopoulos DM, Rigby RA, Akantziliotou C (2004). Instructions on how to use the GAMLSS package in R. Technical Report 02/04. London: STORM Research Centre, London Metropolitan University.

Tanner JM (1952). The assessment of growth and development in children. *Archives of Disease in Childhood*, 27(131):10–33.

Tanner JM, Whitehouse RH, Takaishi M (1966a). Standards from birth to maturity for height, weight, height velocity and weight velocity: British children, 1965. Part I. *Archives of Disease in childhood*, 41:454–71.

Tanner JM, Whitehouse RH, Takaishi M (1966b). Standards from birth to maturity for height, weight, height velocity and weight velocity: British children, 1965. Part II. *Archives of Disease in childhood*, 41:613–35.

Tanner JM, Davies (1985). Clinical longitudinal standards for height and height velocity for North American children. *Journal of Pediatrics*, 107(3):317–29.

van Buuren S, Fredriks M (2001). Worm plot. A simple diagnostic device for modelling growth reference curves. *Statistics in Medicine*, 20:1259–1277.

van't Hof MA, Haschke F, Darvay S (2000). Euro-Growth references on increments in length, weight, head and arm circumferences during the first 3 years of life. Euro-Growth Study Group. *Journal of Pediatric Gastroenterology and Nutrition*, 31 Suppl. 1: S39–47.

WHO Multicentre Growth Reference Study Group (2006a). WHO Child Growth Standards: Length/height-for-age, weight-for-age, weight-for-length, weight-for-height and body mass index-for-age: Methods and development. Geneva: World Health Organization; pp 312 (http://www.who.int/childgrowth/publications/en/, accessed 5 December 2008)

WHO Multicentre Growth Reference Study Group (2006b). Reliability of anthropometric measurements in the WHO Multicentre Growth Reference Study. *Acta Paediatrica*, Suppl. 450:38–46.

WHO Multicentre Growth Reference Study Group (2006c). Enrolment and baseline characteristics in the WHO Multicentre Growth Reference Study. *Acta Paediatrica*, Suppl. 450:7–15.

WHO Multicentre Growth Reference Study Group (2006d). Breastfeeding in the WHO Multicentre Growth Reference Study. *Acta Paediatrica*, Suppl 450:16–26.

WHO Multicentre Growth Reference Study Group (2007). WHO Child Growth Standards: Head circumference-for-age, arm circumference-for-age, triceps skinfold-for-age and subscapular skinfold-for-age: Methods and development. Geneva: World Health Organization; pp 217 (http://www.who.int/childgrowth/publications/en/, accessed 5 December 2008)

WHO Working Group on Infant Growth (1994). An evaluation of infant growth. Geneva: World Health Organization.

WHO (2008). Training course on child growth assessment. Geneva, WHO. (http://www.who.int/childgrowth/training/en/, accessed 5 December 2008).

Wright CM, Matthews JN, Waterston A, Aynsley-Green A (1994). What is a normal rate of weight gain in infancy? *Acta Paediatrica*, 83:351–6.

Wright CM, Avery A, Epstein M, Birks E, Croft D (1998). New chart to evaluate weight faltering. *Archives of Disease in childhood,* 78(1):40-43.

Wright CM (2007). WHO Child Growth Standards: Growth velocity. *Ad hoc Advisory Group meeting on the construction of growth velocity standards.* Geneva, 19-21 March 2007. Background document No. 1.

Appendix B Model specifications of the WHO child growth velocity standards

Table B1 Degrees of freedom for fitting the parameters of the Box-Cox-power exponential (BCPE) distribution for the models with the best fit to generate standards based on age, weight, length, and head circumference in children 0-24 months of age

Standards	Sex	Interval	λ^a	$df(\mu)^b$	$df(\sigma)^c$	$df(v)^d$	τ^e
Weight velocity conditional on age, 0-24 months[f]	Boys	1	0.05	9	4	4	2
		2	0.05	12	6	3	2
		3	0.05	8	3	2	2
		4	0.05	11	5	5	2
		6	0.05	10	5	3	2
	Girls	1	0.05	9	4	1	2
		2	0.05	12	5	4	2
		3	0.05	8	4	4	2
		4	0.05	9	5	5	2
		6	0.05	7	5	4	2
Length velocity conditional on age, 0-24 months	Boys	2	0.05	9	7	1	2
		3	0.05	7	6	1	2
		4	0.05	8	5	1	2
		6	0.05	7	5	1	2
	Girls	2	0.05	10	7	1	2
		3	0.05	8	5	1	2
		4	0.05	8	5	1	2
		6	0.05	7	4	1	2
Head circumference velocity conditional on age, 0-24 months[g]	Boys	2	0.05	8	4	4	2
		3	0.05	7	4	4	2
		4	0.05	10	5	3	2
		6	0.05	9	4	2	2
	Girls	2	0.05	8	4	1	2
		3	0.05	7	4	2	2
		4	0.05	10	5	2	2
		6	0.05	9	5	2	2

[a] Age transformation power
[b] Degrees of freedom for the cubic splines fitting the median (μ)
[c] Degrees of freedom for the cubic splines fitting the coefficient of variation (σ)
[d] Degrees of freedom for the cubic splines fitting the Box-Cox transformation power (v)
[e] Parameter related to the kurtosis fixed ($\tau=2$)
[f] Age range is 0 to 12 months for interval equals to 1
[g] Age range is 0 to 12 months for intervals 2 and 3

Appendix C Results from analyses related to regression to the mean

Table C1 Proportions of children falling below/rising above their starting z-scores (time1) after 1- or 2-month periods (time2)

1-month interval	Starting at -2.5 ≤ z ≤ -1.5			Starting at 1.5 ≤ z ≤ 2.5		
Age (months)	n	prop[a]	mean[b]	n	prop[a]	mean[b]
0-1	42	0.21	0.29	64	0.27	-0.32
1-2	47	0.30	0.17	52	0.42	-0.08
2-3	48	0.48	0.07	48	0.48	-0.03
3-4	50	0.52	0.01	49	0.39	-0.03
4-5	50	0.32	0.10	51	0.39	-0.01
5-6	51	0.45	0.05	42	0.38	-0.05
6-7	56	0.52	-0.02	44	0.45	0.00
7-8	56	0.43	0.05	44	0.55	0.00
8-9	52	0.33	0.07	45	0.40	-0.05
9-10	53	0.34	0.06	50	0.40	-0.05
10-11	48	0.35	0.06	57	0.37	-0.05
11-12	56	0.38	0.06	50	0.44	-0.03

2-month interval	Starting at -2.5 ≤ z ≤ -1.5			Starting at 1.5 ≤ z ≤ 2.5		
Age (months)	n	prop[a]	mean[b]	n	prop[a]	mean[b]
0-2	40	0.13	0.57	65	0.20	-0.62
1-3	48	0.31	0.27	47	0.45	-0.22
2-4	48	0.46	0.16	51	0.33	-0.10
3-5	49	0.45	0.08	47	0.36	-0.03
4-6	52	0.38	0.13	48	0.33	-0.11
5-7	49	0.43	0.08	42	0.40	-0.07
6-8	55	0.44	0.02	45	0.47	-0.05
7-9	57	0.28	0.14	44	0.45	-0.03
8-10	53	0.28	0.12	45	0.31	-0.12
9-11	53	0.47	0.08	51	0.33	-0.09
10-12	47	0.32	0.09	54	0.35	-0.05
12-14	52	0.40	0.07	53	0.30	-0.06
14-16	61	0.36	0.09	54	0.35	-0.08
16-18	57	0.33	0.09	50	0.54	0.00
18-20	50	0.32	0.07	45	0.33	-0.08
20-22	59	0.46	0.00	51	0.41	-0.05
22-24	68	0.50	-0.01	50	0.30	-0.10

[a] Proportion of children who drift farther away from the mean

[b] Average change in z-scores (time2 -time1)

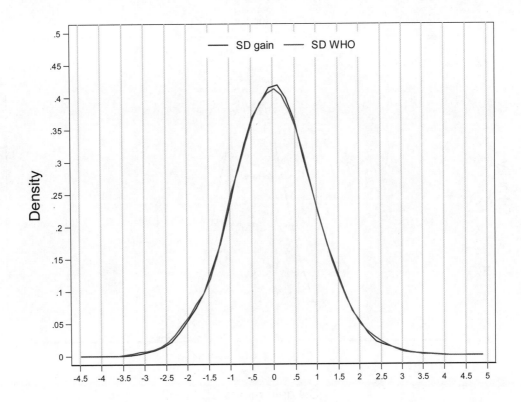

Figure C1 Comparison between 1-month WHO weight increment z-scores and SD$_{gain}$

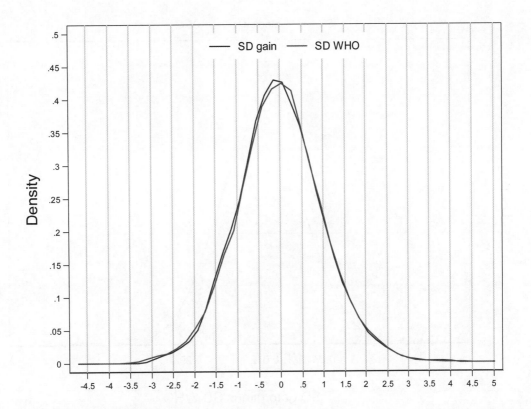

Figure C2 Comparison between 2-month WHO weight increment z-scores and SD$_{gain}$

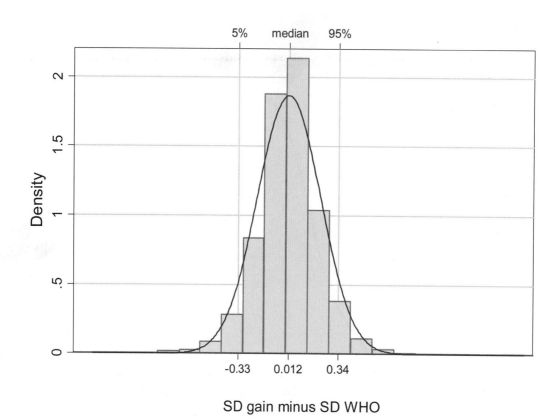

Figure C3 Differences between 1-month WHO weight increment z-scores and SD$_{gain}$

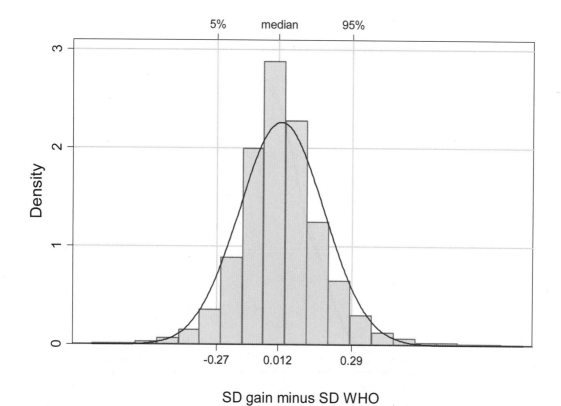

Figure C4 Differences between 2-month WHO weight increment z-scores and SD$_{gain}$